Videos demonstrating step-by-step endoscopic repair of septal perforation are online at MediaCenter.Thieme.com!

	WINDOWS	MAC	TABLET
Recommended Browser(s)**	Recent browser versions on all major platforms and any mobile operating system that supports HTML5 video playback *** all browsers should have JavaScript enabled*		
Flash Player Plug-in	Flash Player 9 or Higher* ** Mac users: ATI Rage 128 GPU does not support full-screen mode with hardware scaling*		Tablet PCs with Android OS support Flash 10.1
Recommended for optimal usage experience	Monitor resolutions: • Normal (4:3) 1024×768 or Higher • Widescreen (16:9) 1280×720 or Higher • Widescreen (16:10) 1440×900 or Higher DSL/Cable internet connection at a minimum speed of 384.0 Kbps or faster WiFi 802.11 b/g preferred.		7-inch and 10-inch tablets on maximum resolution. WiFi connection is required.

Connect with us on social media

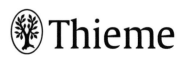

Nasoseptal Perforations: Endoscopic Repair Techniques

Isam Alobid, MD, PhD
Professor
Rhinology and Skull Base Unit
Department of Otolaryngology
Hospital Clinic, University of Barcelona
Barcelona, Spain

Paolo Castelnuovo, MD, FRCSEd, FACS
Full Professor and Chairman
Division of Otorhinolaryngology
Department of Biotechnology and Life Sciences
Head and Neck Surgery & Forensic Dissection Research Center (HNS & FDRC)
University of Insubria
ASST Sette Laghi
Ospedale di Circolo e Fondazione Macchi
Varese, Italy

218 illustrations

Thieme
Stuttgart • New York • Delhi • Rio de Janeiro

Library of Congress Cataloging-in-Publication Data is available from the publisher

© 2017 by Georg Thieme Verlag KG

Thieme Publishers Stuttgart
Rüdigerstrasse 14, 70469 Stuttgart, Germany
+49 [0]711 8931 421, customerservice@thieme.de

Thieme Publishers New York
333 Seventh Avenue, New York, NY 10001 USA
+1 800 782 3488, customerservice@thieme.com

Thieme Publishers Delhi
A-12, Second Floor, Sector-2, Noida-201301
Uttar Pradesh, India
+91 120 45 566 00, customerservice@thieme.in

Thieme Publishers Rio, Thieme Publicações Ltda.
Edifício Rodolpho de Paoli, 25º andar
Av. Nilo Peçanha, 50 – Sala 2508
Rio de Janeiro 20020-906, Brasil
+55 21 3172 2297 / +55 21 3172 1896

Cover design: Thieme Publishing Group
Typesetting by Thomson Digital, India

Printed in India by Replika Press Pvt. Ltd.   5 4 3 2 1

ISBN 978-3-13-205391-5

Also available as an e-book:
eISBN 978-3-13-205401-1

Important note: Medicine is an ever-changing science undergoing continual development. Research and clinical experience are continually expanding our knowledge, in particular our knowledge of proper treatment and drug therapy. Insofar as this book mentions any dosage or application, readers may rest assured that the authors, editors, and publishers have made every effort to ensure that such references are in accordance with **the state of knowledge at the time of production of the book.**

Nevertheless, this does not involve, imply, or express any guarantee or responsibility on the part of the publishers in respect to any dosage instructions and forms of applications stated in the book. **Every user is requested to examine carefully** the manufacturers' leaflets accompanying each drug and to check, if necessary in consultation with a physician or specialist, whether the dosage schedules mentioned therein or the contraindications stated by the manufacturers differ from the statements made in the present book. Such examination is particularly important with drugs that are either rarely used or have been newly released on the market. Every dosage schedule or every form of application used is entirely at the user's own risk and responsibility. The authors and publishers request every user to report to the publishers any discrepancies or inaccuracies noticed. If errors in this work are found after publication, errata will be posted at www.thieme.com on the product description page.

Some of the product names, patents, and registered designs referred to in this book are in fact registered trademarks or proprietary names even though specific reference to this fact is not always made in the text. Therefore, the appearance of a name without designation as proprietary is not to be construed as a representation by the publisher that it is in the public domain.

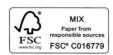

First and foremost, I want to thank my wife, Adriana, and the rest of my family, who supported and encouraged me inspite of all the time it took me away from them. I also want to thank all of the contributors. They made this book worth doing.

Isam Alobid

To my wife Lorella and my sons Matteo, Chiara, Andrea, for making everything possible, for their continued support and love throughout my life.

Paolo Castelnuovo

Contents

Videos

Foreword

When confronted to write a foreword for this book, I wondered whether it was actually needed.

Expanded endonasal approaches (EEA) has raised the need for partial or total reconstruction of the nasal septum to reduce morbidity after surgical removal of skull base tumors during which partial or complete septal resection needed to be carried out to achieve an adequate approach or to reconstruct the skull base defect. Subsequently, septal perforation and aesthetic changes may occur in some cases. Other causes of septal perforations include trauma, surgery, inflammatory or infections, neoplasms, or abuse of inhaled substances.

Thus, on one hand, this topic does not need any introduction. All rhinologists have faced more than one septal defect along their working life, small and larger ones. The first ones were bravely approached surgically, the latter treated with whatever ointments and saline douching to reduce crusting and bleeding. But, so far, no successful surgical approach has guaranteed the closure of perforations that included the total septum or, in other words, when the septum is totally absent. Thus, this book represents a comprehensive overview about the current techniques to achieve close septal perforations and offers an innovative approach to "reconstruct" the full septum that, from my modest point of view, is a surgical revolution. This book comprehensively and completely covers the surgical steps of all the different endoscopic approaches to repair septal perforations. It is a "must" in the libraries of any rhinologist.

On the other hand, I am happy to "introduce" Paolo Castelnuovo, one of the "popes" in Rhinology and Extended Endoscopic Skull Base Surgery. His written contributions are a "must" for those starting in this field—to see how skillfully he dissects in full knowledge of anatomy. It is like watching a wonderful movie.

Isam Alobid established the Skull Base Unit at our Institution some 10 years ago and has pushed himself into the forefront of Rhinology, publishing extraordinary articles and organizing FESS and Skull Base courses since long, thus his name "rings a bell" in our subspecialty since long.

I am sure that both "pioneers" have fulfilled the expectations raised by the title of the book. It is going to become a major success.

Manuel Bernal-Sprekelsen

Preface

Over the past two decades, there has been a dramatic evolution in the manner in which septal perforation repair with endoscopic techniques are approached and managed. Although there are some chapters on external approaches to repair septal defects included in other books about rhinoplasty, there is no book that comprehensively and completely covers the surgical steps of all the different endoscopic approaches to repair septal perforation.

This textbook represents a current state of the art in septal perforation repair. It includes a detailed exposition of the techniques required for complete and successful reconstruction of nasal septum written by many of the world experts who have played an important role in the innovation and expansion of this field.

We believe that this book, with photo series of fresh cadaver dissection, explanatory drawings and correlated radiological images, and short and long follow-up, could be shown to meet the educational and reference needs of the target audiences.

Finally, I would like to express my sincere thanks to all contributors for their excellent contributions and for their willingness to share their fund of experience and knowledge to promote the art and science of septal perforation repair, which reflects positively on the quality of life of the patients whom we serve and to whom we will forever be indebted.

Acknowledgments

The editors would like to acknowledge the help of all the people involved in this project and, more specifically, the contributors who took part in the process. Without their support, this book would not have become a reality. We would like to thank our fellows for their feedback, cooperation, and, of course, friendship. We thank Mr. Stephan Konnry and his team for supporting this project.

Contributors

Juan Ramón Gras Albert, MD, PhD
Professor
Department of Otolaryngology-Head and
  Neck Surgery
Hospital Universitario de Alicante
Universidad Miguel Hernandez
Alicante, Spain

Isam Alobid, MD, PhD
Professor
Rhinology and Skull Base Unit
Department of Otolaryngology
Hospital Clinic, University of Barcelona
Barcelona, Spain

Huseyin Altun, MD
Consultant
Department of ENT
Yunus Emre Hospital
Istanbul, Turkey

Tareck Ayad, MD, FRCSC
Associate Professor
Department of Otolaryngology and Head
  Neck Surgery
Université de Montréal
Montréal, Canada

Leonardo Balsalobre, MD
PhD Student
Department of Otolaryngology and Head
  Neck Surgery
Federal University of Sao Paulo
ENT Center of Sao Paulo
Sao Paulo, Brazil

Ilyes Berania, MD
Consultant
Department of Otolaryngology and Head
  Neck Surgery
Université de Montréal
Montréal, Canada

Eugenio Cárdenas, MD, PhD
Neurosurgeon
Department of Neurosurgery
Hospital Universitario Virgen del Rocío y
  Virgen Macarena
Sevilla, Spain

Michele Cassano, MD
Consultant
Department of ENT
University of Foggia
Foggia, Italy

Paolo Castelnuovo, MD, FRCSEd, FACS
Full Professor and Chairman
Division of Otorhinolaryngology
Department of Biotechnology and Life Sciences
Head and Neck Surgery & Forensic Dissection
  Research Center (HNS & FDRC)
University of Insubria
ASST Sette Laghi
Ospedale di Circolo e Fondazione Macchi
Varese, Italy

Arturo Cordero Castillo, MD
Consultant
Rhinology and Skull Base Unit
Department of Otolaryngology
Hospital Clinic, University of Barcelona
Barcelona, Spain

Mauricio López Chacón, MD
Consultant
Rhinology and Skull Base Unit
Department of Otolaryngology
Hospital Clinic, University of Barcelona
Barcelona, Spain

Giacomo Ceroni Compadretti, MD
Consultant
Department of Otorhinolaryngology
Imola Hospital
Bologna, Italy

Fabio Ferreli, MD
Consultant
Division of Otorhinolaryngology
Department of Biotechnology and Life Sciences
Head and Neck Surgery & Forensic Dissection
  Research Center (HNS & FDRC)
University of Insubria
ASST Sette Laghi
Ospedale di Circolo e Fondazione Macchi
Varese, Italy

Jonathon Frankel, MD
Consultant
MetroHealth Medical Center
Department of Otolaryngology
Case Western Reserve University
Cleveland, Ohio

Elena Garcia-Garrigós, MD
Consultant
Department of Radiology
Hospital Universitario de Alicante
Universidad Miguel Hernandez
Alicante, Spain

Alfonso García-Piñero, MD, PhD
Consultant
Rhinology Unit
ENT Department
HUiP La Fe.
Valencia, Spain

Juan R. Gras-Cabrerizo, MD
Consultant
Department of Otolaryngology-Head and
  Neck Surgery
Hospital de la Santa Creu i Sant Pau
Universitat Autònoma de Barcelona
Barcelona, Spain

Deniz Hanci, MD
Consultant
Department of ENT
Okmeydani Education and Research Hospital
Istanbul, Turkey

Sung Jae Heo, MD
Assistant Professor
Department of Otorhinolaryngology-Head and
  Neck Surgery
Kyungpook National University
School of Medicine
Daegu, Republic of Korea

Steven M Houser, MD, FAAOA
Director of Rhinology, Sinus and Allergy
MetroHealth Medical Center
Department of Otolaryngology
Case Western Reserve University
Cleveland, Ohio

Emily Hrismalos, MD
Consultant
MetroHealth Medical Center
Department of Otolaryngology
Case Western Reserve University
Cleveland, Ohio

Francesca Jaume, MD
Consultant
Rhinology and Skull Base Unit
Department of Otolaryngology
Hospital Clinic, University of Barcelona
Barcelona, Spain

Ariel Kaen, MD, PhD
Neurosurgeon
Department of Neurosurgery
Hospital Universitario Virgen del Rocío y
  Virgen Macarena
Sevilla, Spain

Jung Soo Kim, MD
Professor
Department of Otorhinolaryngology-Head and Neck
  Surgery
Kyungpook National University
School of Medicine
Daegu, Republic of Korea

Cristobal Langdon, MD
Associate Professor
Rhinology and Skull Base Unit
Department of Otolaryngology
Hospital Clinic, University of Barcelona
Barcelona, Spain

Philippe Lavigne, MD
Consultant
Department of Otolaryngology and Head
  Neck Surgery
Université de Montréal
Montréal, Canada

José J. Letort, MD
Professor
Department of ENT
Hospital Metropolitano
Pontificia Universidad Católica del Ecuador
Quito, Ecuador

Paula Mackers, MD
Consultant
Rhinology and Skull Base Unit
Department of Otolaryngology
Hospital Clinic, University of Barcelona
Barcelona, Spain

Hesham A. K. A. Mansour, MD
Professor of Ear, Nose and Throat
Cairo University
Cairo, Egypt

Humbert Massegur-Solench, MD
Consultant
Department of Otolaryngology-Head and
    Neck Surgery
Hospital de la Santa Creu i Sant Pau
Universitat Autònoma de Barcelona
Barcelona, Spain

Meritxell Valls Mateus, MD
Consultant
Department of Otorhinolaryngology
Hospital Clinic, University of Barcelona
Barcelona, Spain

Pietro Palma, MD, FACS
Consultant
Division of Otorhinolaryngology
Department of Biotechnology and Life Sciences
Head and Neck Surgery & Forensic Dissection
    Research Center (HNS & FDRC)
University of Insubria
ASST Sette Laghi
Ospedale di Circolo e Fondazione Macchi
Varese, Italy

Shirley Shizue Nagata Pignatari, MD, PhD
Associate Professor
Division of Pediatric Otolaryngology
Federal University of Sao Paulo
Sao Paulo, Brazil

Alfonso Santamaría, MD
Consultant
Rhinology and Skull Base Unit
Department of Otolaryngology
Hospital Clinic, University of Barcelona
Barcelona, Spain

Juan Antonio Simal-Julian, MD, PhD
Consultant
Endoscopic Skull Base Unit Coordinator
Department of Neurosurgery
HUiP La Fe
Valencia, Spain

Aldo Cassol Stamm, MD, PhD
Affiliated Professor
Department of Otolaryngology and Head and
    Neck Surgery
Federal University of Sao Paulo
Director
ENT Center of Sao Paulo
Sao Paulo, Brazil

Ignazio Tasca, MD
Chief of ENT Department
Department of Otorhinolaryngology
Imola Hospital
Bologna, Italy

Chapter 1

Nasal Anatomy

1

1 Nasal Anatomy

Alfonso García-Piñero, Eugenio Cárdenas, Ariel Kaen, Juan Antonio Simal-Julian

Summary

The nasal cavity is the space comprised in between the external nares and the choanae. In the sagittal axis, this space is divided into two cavities by the nasal septum. In the coronal plane, the nasal cavities extend from the palate to the skull base and from the nasal septum to the lateral nasal wall.

To systematize the surgical endoscopic anatomy of the nose, we approach each nasal cavity as a hexahedron. The anterior and posterior walls of the cube are the nares and the choanae, respectively, the medial wall is the nasal septum, the lateral wall is the homonymous part of the nose, the inferior wall is the nasal floor, and the superior wall is the nasal vault.

The paranasal sinuses are adjacent to these nasal walls. In the roof of the nasal cavity, the frontal sinus, the ethmoidal cells, and the sphenoid sinus are located in an anteroposterior way. The maxillary sinuses are located beside the lateral nasal walls.

The anatomy of the nasal cavity and the paranasal sinuses is exposed/discussed in this chapter in a similar way as an endoscopic approach is performed with respect to the underlying anatomy and each nasal wall.

1.1 Front Door to Nasal Cavity

1.1.1 Piriform Aperture

The piriform aperture acts as the door to the bony structures of the nose. Its boundaries are superiorly the inferior edge of both the nasal bones, laterally the nasal (ascending) processes of the maxilla, and inferiorly the horizontal processes of the maxillary bones. The junction between the latter ones forms the anterior nasal spine, a keel-shaped protrusion in which the nasal septum is firmly attached (► Fig. 1.1).

1.1.2 Nasal Pyramid

The bony framework of the piriform aperture represents the insertion of the cartilaginous structures supporting the nasal pyramid: upper lateral cartilages (ULCs) and lower lateral cartilages (LLCs). The ULCs are triangle shaped. Its superior insertion is under the nasal bones where they are strongly attached. Medially, its edge merges with the nasal septum and the contralateral ULC at the *keystone area* (► Fig. 1.2). This union with the nasal septum shapes a decreasing angle in the nasal cavity from

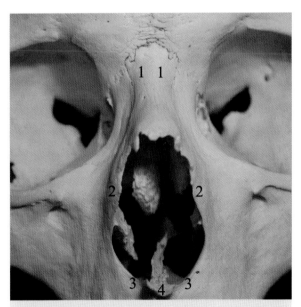

Fig. 1.1 Pyriform aperture.
Skull: 1, nasal bones; 2, ascending processes of the maxilla; 3, horizontal processes of the maxillary bones; 4, anterior nasal spine.

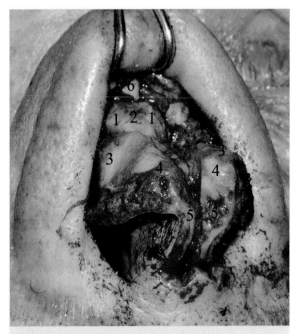

Fig. 1.2 Nasal pyramid.
Open rhinoplasty approach with nasal cartilages exposed: 1, upper lateral cartilages (ULCs); 2, keystone area; 3, cruris lateralis of the lower lateral cartilages (LLCs); 4, domes of the LLC; 5, cruris medialis of the LLC; 6, nasal bones.

superior to inferior (from 70 to 10–15 degrees), which is of paramount importance to determine the nasal airflow. At this point, between the nasal septum, ULC, the head of the middle turbinate, and the floor of the nasal cavity, the coronal section is called "nasal valve" as it constitutes the place of maximal resistance to nasal airflow. Values of this valvular nasal angle under 10 degrees may result in nasal obstruction.[1] The *vertex* of the ULC is inserted laterally in the frontal process of the maxilla. The inferior edge of the ULC is placed under the superior edge of the LLC *crus lateralis*. The LLC is horseshoe shaped and has three portions: *crus medialis*, *crus lateralis*, and intermediate *crus* or *dome*. This cartilage is the main support to the nasal vestibule that is the natural entry to the nasal cavity. Because of its fibroelastic insertions to the bony framework of the piriform aperture and to the musculocutaneous components of the nasal pyramid, it offers a significant elasticity that facilitates the indispensable maneuvers for the endoscopic approaches to the nose.

1.2 Medial Wall of Nasal Cavity: Nasal Septum

The nasal septum is constituted by the septal cartilage and four bones: the perpendicular plate of the ethmoid, the vomer, septal crests of the palatine, and maxillary bones.

Classically the septum was divided by Cottle into five areas, corresponding to the projection of anatomical structures located in the lateral nasal wall: area I, from the external nostril to the nasal valve; area II, corresponding to the nasal valve; area III, from the nasal valve to the anterior limit of the head of the turbinates; area IV, corresponding to the projection of the turbinates; and area V, from the tail of the turbinates to the choana. This classification may be of interest to designate precisely the anatomical location of nasoseptal perforations (▶ Fig. 1.3).

1.2.1 Septal Cartilage

Its anterosuperior edge articulates with the suture between both the nasal bones in the most superior portion; its middle part is the place of insertion of the ULCs of the nasal dorsum and its lower third forms the "supratip" of the nose, being the main support for the nasal tip. The anteroinferior edge hangs just over the *crus medialis* of the LLCs and separated of them by the membranous septum. The posteroinferior edge articulates with the anterior nasal spine, the septal crests of both the maxillary bones (also named *wings of the premaxilla*), and the anterior half of the vomer. Interesting in this area are the fibrous junctions that keep the septal cartilage firmly attached to its inferior bony insertions: direct and crossing fibers from periosteum to perichondrium. The

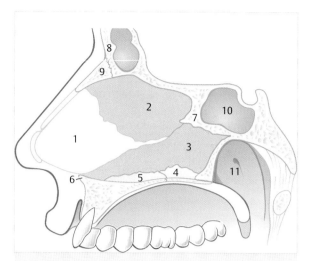

Fig. 1.3 Nasal septum.
Sagittal cut of the head; view of the nasal septum: 1, septal cartilage; 2, perpendicular plate of the ethmoid; 3, vomer; 4, septal crest of the palatine bone; 5, septal crest of the maxilla; 6, anterior nasal spine; 7, rostrum of the sphenoid; 8, frontal bone; 9, nasal bone; 10, sphenoid sinus; 11, eustachian tube.

posterosuperior edge of the cartilage joins the perpendicular plate of the ethmoid in an oblique line from anterior to posterior and superior to inferior. This boundary shows a clear change of consistency between the bone and cartilage when surgically exposed.

1.2.2 Perpendicular Plate of Ethmoid

Its superior edge is inserted in the cribriform plate, where it continues inside the endocranium as the *crista galli*. The anterosuperior edge of the plate is projected forward to articulate with the nasal spine of the frontal bone and the nasal bones. As it has been mentioned, its anteroinferior edge articulates with the septal cartilage. Its inferior edge joins the vomer, often resulting in a bony lateral ridge (▶ Fig. 1.4). In the posterior edge it articulates with the vertical crest located in the middle of the *rostrum sphenoidale*, in between both ostia of the sphenoid sinuses.

1.2.3 Vomer

It has a pointing forward wedge shape. Its posteroinferior edge is the medial limit and the separation of the choanae. Its posterosuperior limit articulates through a V-shaped sulcus with the middle crest of the *rostrum sphenoidale*. Its anterosuperior edge is firmly attached to the perpendicular plate of the ethmoid bone and the septal cartilage. Its inferior edge articulates with the vertical septal crests of the maxillary and palatine bones (see ▶ Fig. 1.3).

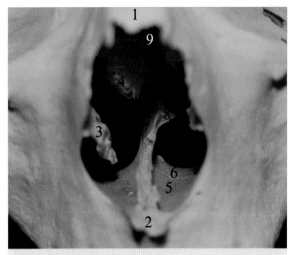

Fig. 1.4 Bony nasal septum.
Skull; bony structures of the nasal cavities: 1, nasal bones; 2, anterior nasal spine; 3, inferior turbinate; 4, middle turbinate; 5; horizontal process of the maxilla; 6, horizontal process or the palatine bone; 7, vomer; 8, bony septal ridge in the joint between perpendicular plate of ethmoid and vomer; 9, posterior edge of the vomer articulating in the *rostrum* of the sphenoid.

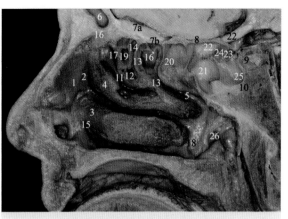

Fig. 1.5 Lateral nasal wall.
Cadaver dissection; right nasal cavity on the sagittal plane. The nasal septum has been removed: 1, lacrimal bulge constituted by the ascending process of the maxilla; 2, lacrimal bone; 3, inferior turbinate; 4, head of the middle turbinate; 5, superior turbinate; 6, frontal sinus; 7a, crista galli; 7b, cribriform plate; 8, planum sphenoidale; 9, sella turcica; 10, clivus; 11, uncinate process; 12, ethmoidal bulla; 13, basal lamella of the middle turbinate (fenestrated); 14, retrobullar recess; 15, drainage of the nasolacrimal duct; 16, lamina papyracea (through the fenestration of the basal lamella); 17, hiatus semilunaris; 18, vertical process of the palatine bone; 19, cells of the anterior ethmoid; 20, cells of the posterior ethmoid; 21, sphenoidal sinus; 22, optic nerve; 23, internal carotid artery (fenestrated); 24, lateral optic-carotid recess; 25, clival recess; 26, eustachian tube.

1.2.4 Septal Crests of Palatine and Maxillary Bones

The septal crests of these two bones form the inferior strip of the nasal septum. They are oriented vertically and join with its contralateral homologous, creating a sulcus where the perpendicular plate of the ethmoid and the septal cartilage are inserted. Often, a septal spur is observed, frequently bilateral, in the line of the joint between the septal cartilage and the septal crest of the maxillary bone, which hinders the subperiosteal-subperichondrial dissection of this area—and even more so because this is the place where the attaching fibers cross from one side to another (see ▸ Fig. 1.4).

1.3 Lateral Nasal Wall

1.3.1 Lateral Wall of Nasal Cavity

We describe the different structures and reliefs that will be found in the endoscopic exploration from anterior to posterior (▸ Fig. 1.5).

Frontal Process of Maxillary Bone

The anterior edge of the frontal or ascending process of the maxillary bone forms the piriform aperture in its lower part and articulates with the nasal bones superiorly. Its superior limit joins the frontal bone. Its medial surface is the most anterior part of the lateral wall of the nose and presents two horizontal crests for the insertion of the inferior and the middle turbinates. The posterior edge of the frontal process articulates with the lacrimal bone and forms what is endoscopically known as *maxillary crest* or *lacrimal bulge*, a vertical relief of thick bone that is covering medially the lacrimal sac (▸ Fig. 1.6).

Lacrimal Bone

The lacrimal bone (also known as *unguis*) is a quadrangular, usually thin bone located posterior to the lacrimal bulge and anterior to the lamina papyracea of the ethmoid. It goes from the frontal bone superiorly to the inferior turbinate inferiorly. Its lateral surface has a vertical crest dividing it into a posterior sulcus corresponding to the orbital wall and *agger nasi* and an anterior one that forms the nasolacrimal duct.

Nasolacrimal Duct

The nasolacrimal duct runs downward and drains the content of the lacrimal sac. The route of the duct starts at the medial orbital wall, runs to the inferior meatus, and ends in this meatus just under the head of the inferior turbinate. Precautions should be taken when harvesting reconstructive mucosal flaps from the nasal lateral wall to avoid damaging this duct. The medial wall of the duct

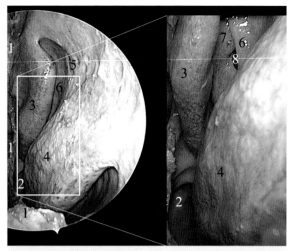

Fig. 1.6 Middle meatus.
Cadaver dissection; left nasal cavity; nasal septum detached (endoscopic view). In the enlargement the middle meatus is medialized: 1, nasal septum; 2, left choana; 3, middle turbinate; 4, inferior turbinate; 5, lacrimal bulge; 6, uncinate process; 7, ethmoidal bulla; 8, ostium of the maxillary sinus.

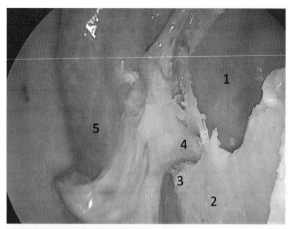

Fig. 1.7 Sphenopalatine artery.
Left nasal cavity (endoscopic view). The maxillary sinus has been wide opened: 1, posterior wall of maxillary sinus; 2, vertical process of palatine bone; 3, ethmoidal crest (pointer); 4, sphenopalatine artery (turbinal branch); 5, tail of the middle turbinate.

is formed by the lacrimal bone and the inferior turbinate. Its lateral wall is the frontal process of the maxilla.

Agger Nasi Cells

The *agger nasi* is the most anterior part of the ethmoid. In the endoscopic examination it is seen as a prominence of the lateral nasal wall, anterior to the attachment of the middle turbinate[2] (see ▶ Fig. 1.5). Its pneumatization is highly variable and it may narrow the frontal recess considerably.

Inferior Turbinate

This independent bone has a rounded and slightly elongated shape, like a shell, and is attached to the lateral wall of the nose by means of three processes: the lacrimal process, which articulates with the inferior turbinal crest of the frontal process of the maxilla; the ethmoidal process, which articulates with the uncinate process; and the maxillary process, which contours the inferior boundary of the maxillary sinus ostium.

Middle Turbinate

In a sagittal plane, the anterior third of the middle turbinate can be attached superiorly in most cases to the skull base between the cribriform plate and the lateral lamella of the ethmoid. Its medial surface is oriented to the nasal septum and its lateral surface to the middle meatus.

When this portion of the turbinate is pneumatized (15–50%), it is called *concha bullosa*.[3]

The middle third of the turbinate or *basal lamella* is placed in a coronal plane but inclined from top to bottom anteroposteriorly. It is inserted in the *lamina papyracea* and separates the anterior from the posterior ethmoidal cells.

The posterior third is mostly horizontal, and its insertion in the *lamina papyracea* and in the ethmoidal crest of the vertical process of the palatine bone delimits the area where the sphenopalatine artery enters the nasal cavity (▶ Fig. 1.7).

Uncinate Process

It is a very thin bony structure with the shape of the bow of a sled's runner. Its anterior portion is vertically oriented and its posterior one is horizontal, running in the sagittal plane. The anterosuperior end attaches in more than a half of cases in the lamina papyracea although six different types of insertion have been described,[4] including to the middle turbinate or the skull base. Its posteroinferior end usually articulates with the ethmoidal process of the inferior turbinate and the vertical process of the palatine bone. Anteriorly it is attached to the lacrimal bone and its posterior edge is usually free, leading to the inferior semilunar hiatus, between the ethmoidal bulla and the uncinate process. The lateral surface constitutes the medial limit of the ethmoidal infundibulum (see ▶ Fig. 1.6).

Perpendicular Plate of Palatine Bone

Its anterior edge contributes to close the aperture of the maxillary sinus in the posterior limit of the maxillary ostium. In the medial surface the crests for the insertion of the middle and inferior turbinates are observed. Its posterior edge continues with the medial plate of the pterygoid process of the sphenoid. Its superior edge consists of the sphenoidal and orbital process with in between the sphenopalatine foramen, just beneath the sphenoid. The anterior rim of this foramen, containing the sphenopalatine vessels and nasopalatine nerve, is observed endoscopically as a ridge known as *ethmoidal crest* (see ▶ Fig. 1.7).

1.3.2 Maxillary Sinus

The maxillary sinus has an inverted pyramid shape. The medial wall of the maxillary sinus is made up by the lateral wall of the nose. If the bones of the nasal lateral wall are removed, the remaining is a large bony orifice formerly known as *Highmore's antrum*. This orifice is reduced to a smaller size by means of the lacrimal bone, the uncinate process, the inferior turbinate, the vertical process of the palatine bone, and the ethmoid cells (see ▶ Fig. 1.5). Projecting into the floor of the sinus, there are several conical processes, corresponding to the roots of the first and second molar teeth. The roof of the sinus is formed by the floor of the orbit, and it is crossed from posterior to anterior by the infraorbital nerve and vessel. The posterior wall of the sinus separates the antrum from the pterygopalatine fossa medially and the infratemporal fossa laterally.

1.4 Ceiling of Nasal Cavity: Nasal Vault, Ethmoid Cells, and Frontal Sinus

The roof of the nasal cavity is constituted by four bones: the nasal bones, the frontal bone, the ethmoid, and the sphenoid. The insertion of the middle turbinate in the skull base separates the superior wall in a medial and lateral part called *the cribriform plate* and the *fovea ethmoidalis*, respectively (▶ Fig. 1.8).

The anterior limits of the cribriform plate are the inferior part of the frontal bone (frontal beak) and the posterosuperior edge of the nasal bone. The olfactory fibers pass through the cribriform plate from the olfactory fossa to the olfactory cleft. The lateral limit consists of the medial surface of the middle turbinate and the medial limit of the upper third of the nasal septum, corresponding to the middle turbinate. The cribriform plate ends posteriorly in the anterior wall of the sphenoid bone (*rostrum sphenoidale*), leaving the sphenoethmoidal recess between the superior turbinate and the nasal septum, where the natural ostium of the sphenoid sinus is located[5] (▶ Fig. 1.9).

The lateral lamella of the ethmoidal plate extends laterally and upward in the cribriform plate. The height of the lateral lamella (and the depth of the olfactory cleft therefore) has been classified by Keros into three types: type 1 (1–3 mm), type 2 (4–7 mm), and type 3 (8–16 mm),[6] and it usually decreases from anterior to posterior[7] (see ▶ Fig. 1.8).

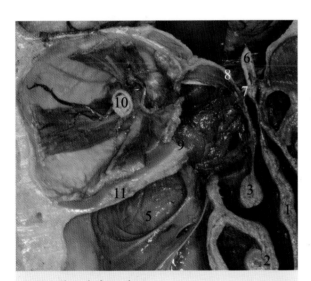

Fig. 1.8 The cribriform plate.
Cadaver dissection; coronal cut through the right orbit: 1, nasal septum; 2, inferior turbinate; 3, middle turbinate; 4, basal lamella of the middle turbinate (once anterior ethmoidal cells resected); 5, maxillary sinus; 6, crista galli; 7, cribriform plate; 8, lateral lamella; 9, lamina papyracea (resected); 10, optic nerve; 11, infraorbitary nerve.

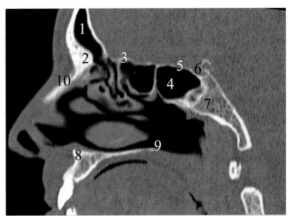

Fig. 1.9 Nasal vault.
CT scan, sagittal view: 1, frontal sinus; 2, "beak" of the frontal bone; 3, cribriform plate of the ethmoid; 4, sphenoid sinus; 5, planum sphenoidale; 6, sella turcica; 7, clivus; 8, anterior nasal spine; 9, posterior nasal spine; 10, nasal bones.

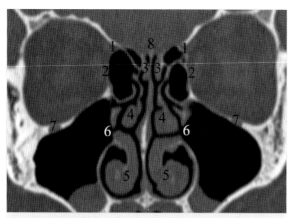

Fig. 1.10 Anterior ethmoidal arteries.
CT scan, coronal plane: 1, anterior ethmoidal arteries; 2, lamina papyracea; 3, superior turbinate; 4, middle turbinate; 5 inferior turbinate; 6, maxillary ostium; 7, infraorbital nerve; 8, crista galli.

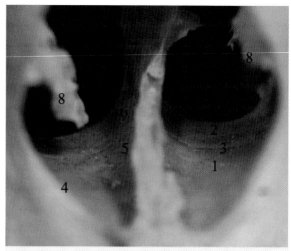

Fig. 1.11 Nasal floor.
Skull, bony structures of the nasal cavities, anterior view: 1, palatine process of the maxilla; 2, horizontal process of the palatine bone; 3, cruciform suture; 4, pyriform aperture; 5, septal crest of the maxilla; 6, septal crest of the palatine bone; 7, vomer; 8 inferior turbinates.

1.4.1 Ethmoid Cells

Between the middle and superior turbinate medially and the lamina papyracea laterally lies the ethmoidal complex, which is divided by the basal lamella of the middle turbinate into the anterior ethmoid and posterior ethmoid (▶ Fig. 1.9). The ethmoidal bulla is the largest anterior ethmoidal cell and its anterior surface forms the posterior border of the semilunar hiatus (between bulla and uncinate process). The ethmoidal infundibulum is located between lamina papyracea and uncinate process, and the frontal recess between bulla, lamina papyracea, and agger nasi. The retrobullar recess lies between the posterior face of bulla ethmoidalis and the basal lamella when both are separated. The suprabullar recess is formed when the bulla does not reach the ethmoidal roof, between the bulla and the frontal recess. It is the most common site to find the anterior ethmoidal artery, traversing the ethmoidal roof from posterolateral to anteromedial[7] (▶ Fig. 1.10). The posterior ethmoid comprises a number of inconstant cells distributed from the basal lamella to the rostrum sphenoidale and from the lamina papyracea to the superior turbinate. Just to mention is the Onodi's cell that can enter into the sphenoid bone and encircle the optic nerve. The posterior ethmoidal artery usually crosses within the ethmoidal roof in this area, just before the superior aspect of the *rostrum sphenoidale*.

The ostiomeatal complex is a functional concept that comprises the drainage pathways of the middle meatus, the anterior ethmoidal complex, suprabullar and frontal recesses, and ethmoidal infundibulum (see ▶ Fig. 1.6).

1.4.2 Frontal Sinus

The frontal recess is accepted to be the most anterosuperior part of the ethmoid, just inferior to the frontal sinus opening and superomedial to the agger nasi cells. Its posterior limit is the anterior wall of the ethmoidal bulla; laterally it is limited by the lamina papyracea and inferiorly with the vertex of the ethmoidal infundibulum.

Between the frontal recess and the frontal sinus, a series of pneumatized cells could be seen extending from the agger nasi, ethmoidal bulla, or terminal recess of the ethmoidal infundibulum. They are called *anterior ethmoidal cells* if they do not extend into the frontal sinus or *frontoethmoidal cells* if they do so.

The frontal sinus opening is located in the lower part of the sinus and it may be drained by an ostium or an infundibulum. The pneumatization of this sinus is very variable, and considerable variations in shape, size, and position of intersinus septum and other secondary septations can be found[8] (see ▶ Fig. 1.5).

1.5 Nasal Floor

It is slightly concave transversely and has a smooth surface, which facilitates the harvesting of reconstructive mucoperiosteal flaps. It consists of both the palatine process of the maxilla and the horizontal process of the palatine bone (▶ Fig. 1.11).

1.5.1 Palatine Process of Maxilla

The anterior limit is the lower part of the rim of the piriform aperture, which has an anteriorly ascending orientation. The medial edge, in a vertical disposition, articulates with its contralateral homonymous at the septal crest. Right behind the medial piriform crest and the anterior nasal spine, there are the inlet orifices of the anterior

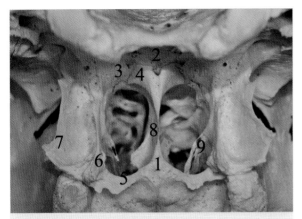

Fig. 1.12 Choanae.
Skull, bony structures of the choanae, posterior view: 1, posterior nasal spine; 2, body of the sphenoid; 3, sphenoidal process of palatine bone; 4, wing of the vomer; 5, horizontal process of palatine bone; 6, medial plate of the pterygoid; 7, lateral plate of the pterygoid; 8, vomer; 9, inferior turbinate.

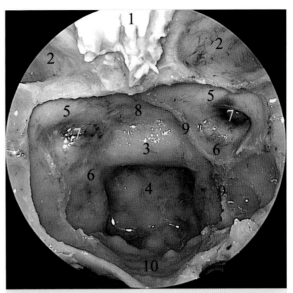

Fig. 1.13 Sphenoid sinus.
Cadaver dissection, the rostrum sphenoidale has been resected and both sphenoidal sinuses communicated (endoscopic view): 1, nasal septum; 2, posterosuperior ethmoidal cells; 3, sella turcica; 4, clival recess; 5, optic nerves; 6, bulges of internal carotid arteries; 7, lateral optic-carotid recesses; 8, planum sphenoidale; 9; intersinus septum (note the insertion of the septum towards the left carotid artery); 10, floor of the sinus.

palatine duct (for the nasopalatine vessels and nerves). The posterior edge of the process articulates with the anterior edge of the horizontal process of the palatine bone by means of a suture (cruciform) that is virtually unappreciable from an endoscopic view.

1.5.2 Horizontal Process of Palatine Bone

The limit not described previously is its posterior edge that forms the inferior rim of the choana, where the muscles of the soft palate are inserted. The joint of both horizontal processes forms the posterior nasal spine (▶ Fig. 1.12).

1.6 Back Door of Nasal Cavity

1.6.1 Choana

The choana has a quadrilateral shape with rounded corners. The superior boundary is the body of the sphenoid bone. The medial boundary is covered by the sphenoidal process of the palatine bone laterally and the wings of the vomer medially, inferiorly the horizontal process of the palatine bone, laterally the vertical process of the palatine bone and its joint with the medial plate of the pterygoid process, and medially the vomer (see ▶ Fig. 1.12).

1.6.2 Sphenoid Sinus

The sphenoid sinus constitutes the arch of the choana. Just on top, the body of the sphenoid bone is located. The pneumatization of this body forms the two sphenoid sinuses, frequently asymmetric in size and separated by an intersinus septum (medial wall of the sinus). The

intersinus septum is attached to the rostrum of the *sella turcica* or often, more laterally, to the internal carotid artery or the optic nerve tubercles. Additionally, partial septations are frequently encountered. Depending on the degree of pneumatization, the form of the sinus has been classified in agenesic, conchal, presellar, and sellar.[9] Another classification has been proposed according to the direction of pneumatization: sphenoid body, lateral clival, lesser wing, anterior into the rostrum, and combined.[10] The anterior wall of both sphenoid sinuses communicates with their respective nasal cavity through the *ostia sphenoidale*, endoscopically observable in the medial portion of the sphenoid *rostrum*, next to the bony nasal septum, and 15 to 20 mm above the arch of the choana. The posterior nasal artery crosses under this ostium from lateral to medial and could be damaged in the inferior endoscopic surgical enlargement of the ostium. The floor of the sinus may be edged by the protrusion of the pterygoid canal containing the Vidian nerve. The lateral wall of the sphenoid sinus is the medial limit of the cavernous sinus, and the protrusion of the third, fourth, fifth (first and second branches), and sixth cranial nerves could be seen. This wall is elevated in the posterior part over the optic nerve canal and the internal carotid artery, from top to floor, and the recess created between both is called *lateral optic-carotid recess*. In the posterior wall of the sinus protrudes the sellar rostrum and below it, depending on the degree of pneumatization of the sphenoid bone, is located the clival recess. Going from the back to the front in the roof of the sinus, the *tuberculum sellae* separates the pituitary fossa from the prechiasmatic sulcus, which is the projection of the optic chiasm (or chiasma opticum); above this sulcus the *limbus sphenoidale* sets the transition from vertical to horizontal: from the location of the chiasma in the sulcus to the *planum sphenoidale*[11] (▶ Fig. 1.13).

References

[1] Méndez-Benegassi I, Maranillo E, Sañudo J. Anatomía de la nariz y de las fosas nasales. In: Suárez C, Gil-Carcedo L, Marco J, Medina J, Ortega P, Trinidad J, eds. Tratado de Otorrinolaringología Y Cirugía de Cabeza Y Cuello. 2nd ed. Madrid, Spain: Editorial Médica Panamericana, SA; 2007:437–463

[2] Stammberger H, Lund V. Anatomy of the nose and paranasal sinuses. In: Gleeson M, Browning G, Burton M, eds. Scott-Brown's Otorhinolaryngology, Head and Neck Surgery. 7th ed. London, UK: Hodder Arnold; 2008:1315–1343

[3] Hatipoğlu HG, Cetin MA, Yüksel E. Concha bullosa types: their relationship with sinusitis, ostiomeatal and frontal recess disease. Diagn Interv Radiol. 2005; 11(3):145–149

[4] Isobe M, Murakami G, Kataura A. Variations of the uncinate process of the lateral nasal wall with clinical implications. Clin Anat. 1998; 11 (5):295–303

[5] Kim HU, Kim SS, Kang SS, Chung IH, Lee JG, Yoon JH. Surgical anatomy of the natural ostium of the sphenoid sinus. Laryngoscope. 2001; 111 (9):1599–1602

[6] Keros P. [On the practical value of differences in the level of the lamina cribrosa of the ethmoid]. Z Laryngol Rhinol Otol. 1962; 41:809–813

[7] Lund VJ, Stammberger H, Fokkens WJ, et al. European position paper on the anatomical terminology of the internal nose and paranasal sinuses. Rhinol Suppl. 2014(24):1–34

[8] Martins C, de Alencastro L, Capel A, et al. Anatomy of the nasal cavity and paranasal sinuses. In: Stamm A, ed. Transnasal Endoscopic Skull Base and Brain Surgery. Tips and Pearls. 1st ed. New York, NY: Thieme Medical Publishers; 2012:15–35

[9] Elwany S, Elsaeid I, Thabet H. Endoscopic anatomy of the sphenoid sinus. J Laryngol Otol. 1999; 113(2):122–126

[10] Wang J, Bidari S, Inoue K, Yang H, Rhoton A, Jr. Extensions of the sphenoid sinus: a new classification. Neurosurgery. 2010; 66(4):797–816

[11] Cárdenas E. Orbitotomía superomedial: nuevos límites en el abordaje endonasal expandido transetmoidal. Doctoral thesis. Spain: Universitat de València; 2015

Chapter 2
Nasal Physiology

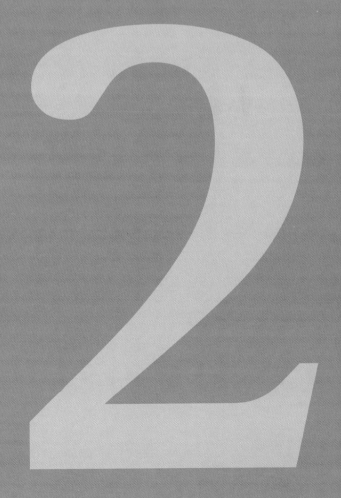

2 Nasal Physiology

Jonathan Frankel, Emily Hrisomalos, Steven M. Houser

Summary

Septal perforation repair is no easy task for the surgeon. A thorough understanding of the tissue involved in the surgical area is essential for proper approach and healing. This chapter serves as a foundation for the surgeon to further such knowledge. The mucosal blanket, including proper and abnormal function, is important to understand, as well as ways to assess nasal function. The authors discuss normal and abnormal nasal physiology as well as how to measure nasal physiology.

2.1 Normal Nasal Physiology
2.1.1 Mucous Blanket and Mucociliary Clearance

Nasal mucosa functions to protect the lower airways from inhalation of particular matter, pathogens, and allergens through both barrier and biochemical protective mechanisms. The pseudostratified ciliated columnar epithelium of the nasal airway, also referred to as *respiratory epithelium*, is made up of ciliated and nonciliated columnar cells, goblet cells, and basal cells. This epithelium is found in the posterior two-thirds of the nasal cavity (posterior to the limen nasi) and produces a mucous blanket both characteristic and vital to function of the upper respiratory tract (▶ Fig. 2.1).[1]

Particle characteristics including size, shape, and aerodynamic qualities determine the degree of deposition. Particles smaller than 0.5 μm will make it past the filter of the nasal airways and into the lower respiratory system. Larger particles are trapped within the multiple filtering mechanisms of the nasal airway. Of particles 1 μm in size, studies have shown that approximately 60% will be deposited in the nasal cavities. This percentage increases further with increasing particle size.[1] Multiple studies have looked at the distribution of caught particles within the nasal cavity, and a site of concentrated deposition has been found to be just posterior to the nasal valve and the anterior aspect of the middle turbinate. The internal valve is the site of transition of airflow from laminar to turbulent after which the flow is directed posteriorly toward the middle turbinate.

Mucin production by goblet cells must be appropriately regulated. Inadequate production can lead to impaired trapping of particles for clearance, whereas overproduction can lead to airway obstruction and impair clearance that can ultimately promote recurrent and persistent respiratory infections. This epithelium lies over a basement membrane that unique to its location in the nasal cavity is permeated by capillaries, which allows fluid to pass directly through these vessels onto the mucosal surface and alter its consistency.[2]

The mucous blanket is driven by ciliary movement toward the lateral pharyngeal walls towards the esophageal inlet for swallowing. Cilia beat at a frequency of 1,000 strokes per minute and the mean velocity of particle transport are estimated at 6 mm/min under normal physiologic conditions.[3] Mucous flow is a barrier to microorganisms, irritants, and allergens. The mucous blanket is described as having two separate layers, the inner, or sol, layer that is thin and driven forward by the beating cilia that it surrounds, and the outer gel layer that is viscous and rich in glycoproteins. This thin inner layer surrounds the cilia and propels the overlying viscous layer posteriorly over its surface. The mucous blanket exits the nasal cavity and is replaced by fresh mucous secretions every 10 to 15 minutes via the activity of this ciliary movement.[3,4]

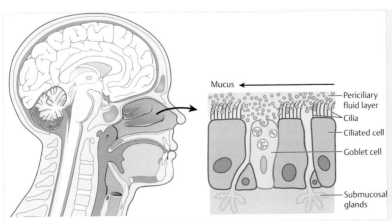

Mucus — Periciliary fluid layer — Cilia — Ciliated cell — Goblet cell — Submucosal glands

Fig. 2.1 Schematic of nasal mucosa.

2.1.2 Innate Mucosal Immunity

Tight junctions and secretions produced by the respiratory epithelium of the nose provide mechanical protection from pathogens and debris.[5,6] These foreign materials are typically cleared by respiratory cilia. However, when the physical defenses provide insufficient protection, the nasal cavity relies on an inflammatory reaction. Innate mucosal immunity is composed of trigger molecules such as toll-like receptors that recognize pattern-associated molecular patterns present on pathogens.[6] The activation of toll-like receptors triggers cytokine release with subsequent induction of the adaptive immune response, as well as the production of nitric oxide (NO).[6] Antimicrobial peptides, including defensins and cathelicidins, are then activated to directly kill bacteria, viruses, and fungi, and further potentiate tissue inflammation.[6,7] Innate mucosal immunity is important especially when the nasal mucosa is physiologically abnormal and cannot clear foreign substances through ciliary clearance.

2.1.3 Nasal Sensation/Innervation

The mimetic muscles covering the external nose are innervated by the facial nerve while its sensory function is provided by branches from the ophthalmic and maxillary divisions of the trigeminal nerve. Sensation of the nasal cavity and septum is provided largely by the maxillary division of the trigeminal nerve, namely the nasopalatine nerve, anterior ethmoidal branch of the nasociliary nerve, as well as the anterior superior alveolar nerve.[1] Branches of the maxillary division have free nerve endings diffusely within the nasal mucosa, which also provides the sensory input from inhalation of irritants that may reflexively lead to protective mechanisms such as sneezing, tearing, or increased secretions.[8] Also important to note is the contribution of autonomic control on nasal blood flow. Sympathetic stimulation leads to reduction in blood flow and decongestion whereas parasympathetic activity increases blood flow and congestion.[1]

2.1.4 Nasal Airflow

Inspired air flows across the nasal mucosa that is thus exposed to a varying amount of particulate matter. The intricate and tortuous anatomy of the nasal cavity serves to increase the surface area available for this exposure, which optimizes olfaction, heating, humidification, and filtering of the inspired air. Airflow reaches its maximum velocity when passing through the internal nasal valve at which point collapse may be seen to varying degrees based on Bernoulli's theorem of airflow showing increased velocity and decreased transmural pressure at areas of reduced caliber.[4,8,9]

Turbulence further increases contact of the estimated 14,000 L of inspired air that on average passes through the nasal cavity, with the nasal mucosa.[8,10]

The nasal cycle, first described by Kayser in 1895, has been shown to be present in approximately 80% of the population. The cycle refers to changes in airway resistance and in nasal passage caliber that alter nasal airflow; submucosal vascular engorgement on one side balances with decongestion on the other side. The cycle occurs every 0.5 to 3 hours.[11] During changes leading to cyclically altered cross-sectional area, the overall combined nasal airway resistance importantly remains unchanged. At times, the nasal cycle may lead to near total obstruction, both subjectively and on clinical and radiologic examination. This comes into play when examining patients reporting nasal obstruction.[4]

Importantly, nasal airflow is also affected by postural changes, exertion, and sex hormones. NO, acting as a neurotransmitter, also significantly contributes to changes in nasal airflow, ciliary beat frequency, and mucous production. Increased airflow leads to a decreased NO concentration in the nasal cavity, an increased NO concentration in the lower respiratory tract, and decreased ciliary beat frequency.[1]

2.2 Abnormal Nasal Physiology

2.2.1 Disorders of Mucociliary Transport

There are a wide range of both congenital and acquired etiologies of mucociliary transport dysfunction. Ciliary dysfunction can be inherited as in primary ciliary dyskinesia (PCD). In PCD, ciliary beating is reduced or absent, resulting in impairment of the mucociliary escalator.[12] Patients with cystic fibrosis have normal ciliary function and structure, but abnormalities in the cystic fibrosis transmembrane conductance regulator result in dysfunctional sodium and chloride transport and subsequent dehydration of the pericellular liquid. In this dehydrated environment, ciliary function is challenged by increased mucous viscosity, and cilia are unable to sufficiently clear debris and infectious pathogens.[13]

2.2.2 Infection and Inflammation

Infective agents and environmental exposures can also interfere with mucociliary transport. For example, the inflammatory edema seen in acute rhinosinusitis impairs normal nasal airflow and limits drainage from the sinus ostium.[14] Edema can thus create an environment in which mucous is stagnant, and debris and pathogens cannot be cleared efficiently. Viruses are typically the inciting pathogens of rhinosinusitis. The most common viral causes of rhinosinusitis include rhinovirus, coronavirus, influenza virus, respiratory syncytial virus, and parainfluenza virus.[15] The ensuing vasodilation and increased vascular permeability from viral infection result in nasal obstruction and rhinorrhea.[15] Decreased clearance of other pathogens may complicate the patient's course with the development of a bacterial rhinosinusitis.[16,17,18] Typically, the predominant bacteria responsible are *Streptococcus pneumoniae, Haemophilus influenzae,* or *Moraxella catarrhalis.*[18] More recently *Staphylococcus aureus* is thought to contribute to acute infections in about 8 to 11% of cases.[19] Fungal infections should also be considered as a potential initiating or contributing pathogen.

2.2.3 Exposure to Ciliotoxic Agents

Drugs administered both systemically and locally in the nose have been found to have ciliotoxic effects, such as β-blockers, local anesthetics, antihistamines, and lipophilic preservatives added to nasal medications.[20] These agents limit cilia's clearance of debris, allergens, and pathogens, and can compromise this very important defensive mechanism. On the other hand, some pharmaceuticals such as cholinergic drugs and β-adrenergic drugs can actually stimulate ciliary function.[20]

It is of no surprise that exposure to various environmental agents can inhibit normal ciliary function as well. Tobacco smoke, in particular, has detrimental effects on ciliary clearance through multiple mechanisms. Tobacco smoke is directly ciliotoxic; it increases mucous production through goblet cell hyperplasia and results in activation of an inflammatory cascade within the respiratory tract.[21]

2.3 Tests of Nasal Physiology

2.3.1 Rhinomanometry

Rhinomanometry is the most commonly used objective measurement of nasal airflow. Airflow is measured at a fixed pressure differential using a pressure sensor. The site of sensor placement, at the contralateral anterior naris versus the nasopharynx, distinguishes anterior from posterior techniques, respectively. In another technique called *postnasal rhinomanometry*, the sensor is placed in the oropharynx and measures the combined nasal resistance of both passages. Airflow within the tested side is measured by a flow sensor contained within a facemask. Results are in the form of a pressure-flow curve. These tests are most commonly performed as active measurements, meaning that the measurements taken are of the patient's own respiratory effort; however, there are also passive tests that are driven by a respiratory pump.[22]

2.3.2 Acoustic Rhinometry

Acoustic rhinometry, developed in 1989 by Hilberg et al, allows for plotting of a two-dimensional profile of the endonasal anatomy through generation of sound wave reflections, thereby allowing for assessment of intranasal volume or cross-sectional area.[22] Acoustic waves are sent into the nasal cavities through an anterior nose piece and reflect back to a microphone after contacting intranasal structures. Results are displayed in graphic form in terms of distances from the nosepiece. Two distinct areas of interest are notches representing the valve angle and the anterior head of the inferior turbinate. As expected, level of nasal congestion significantly influences these measurements. Important to recall is Poiseuille's law that states that airflow is directly proportional to the fourth power of the radius illustrating that seemingly minimal changes in nasal cavity caliber can profoundly affect airflow.[23] Variations of 10 to 16% in the same patient have been indicating relative reproducibility.[4] Results have been correlated with radiologic studies and shown to be most accurate in measuring the anterior nasal cavities, particularly the nasal valve.[23]

2.3.3 Mucociliary Transport

Mucociliary transport can be measured in vivo with a variety of clinical tests. These tests have a high degree of sensitivity and can be used to rule out PCD. However, they have a relatively low specificity, and abnormal results should be followed with further investigation. The saccharine test involves the measurement of time it takes for saccharine placed on the anterior head of the inferior turbinate to be tasted by the patient. Nasal endoscopy can supplement this test by dyeing the saccharine with methylene blue and watching as the saccharine migrates.[24,25] Radioactive technetium-99 m (^{99m}Tc) particles can also be placed on the inferior turbinate or nasal septum and followed by a gamma-camera to identify the time it takes for radioactivity to be cleared from the nasal cavity.[26] Nuclear testing for mucociliary transport is more expensive and performed at a limited number of institutions.[27] Ciliary activity can be studied in vitro as well by looking at biopsied nasal mucosa under phase-contrast microscopy, evaluating presence, and coordination of ciliary movements.[27]

2.3.4 Ciliary Activity

The function of cilia can similarly be studied both in vivo and in vitro. Laser light scattering spectroscopy can directly study the frequency and synchrony of cilia movement by measuring the Doppler effect of scattered light.[28] Brushings or biopsies of cilia typically taken from the inferior or middle turbinates can be studied using high-speed photometry to quantify the ciliary beat frequency.[27] Nasal NO measurement is a noninvasive technique that may suggest PCD, but it has a relatively low sensitivity and specificity.[27] In addition, genetic analysis and evaluation of cell cultures do not directly measure ciliary activity, but they can be used to detect PCD.[27]

2.4 Conclusion

Nasal physiology is a complex interplay between active mucosal elements. Aberrations in mucosal function can occur, and these can be studied through various tests. A thorough understanding of nasal physiology will benefit the surgeon as he/she prepares to undertake repairing a septal perforation.

References

[1] Van Cauwenberge P, Sys L, De Belder T, Watelet JB. Anatomy and physiology of the nose and the paranasal sinuses. Immunol Allergy Clin North Am. 2004; 24(1):1–17

[2] Munzel M. The permeability of intercellular spaces of the nasal mucosa. J Laryngol Rhinol Otol. 1974; 51:794–798

[3] Ganesan S, Comstock AT, Sajjan US. Barrier function of airway tract epithelium. Tissue Barriers. 2013; 1(4):e24997

[4] Boek WM, Graamans K, Natzijl H, van Rijk PP, Huizing EH. Nasal mucociliary transport: new evidence for a key role of ciliary beat frequency. Laryngoscope. 2002; 112(3):570–573

[5] Abbas AK, Lichtman A, Pillai S. Specialized Immunity at Epithelial Barriers and in Immune Privileged Tissues. Cellular and Molecular Immunology. 8th ed. Elsevier; 2015

[6] Baroody FM, Naclerio RM. Allergy and immunology of the upper airway. Cummings Otolaryngology 2014;38:593–625.e10

[7] Dieffenback CW, Tramont EC, Plaeger SF. Innate (general or nonspecific) host defense mechanisms. Mandell, Douglas, and Bennett's Principles and Practice of Infectious Diseases. Vol. 4. Saunders (an imprint of Elsevier); 2015:26–33.e2

[8] Jones N. The nose and paranasal sinuses physiology and anatomy. Adv Drug Deliv Rev. 2001; 51(1–3):5–19

[9] Kern EB. Surgery of the Face and Neck: Proceedings of the Second International Symposium. Vol. 2. New York, NY: Grune and Stratton; 1977:43–59

[10] Cole P. Modification of inspired air. In: Proctor DR, Andersen I, eds. The Nose, Upper Airway Physiology, and the Atmospheric Environment. Amsterdam, The Netherlands: Elsevier Biomedical Press; 1982:351–375

[11] Eccles R. Nasal airflow in health and disease. Acta Otolaryngol. 2000; 120(5):580–595

[12] Bush A, Chodhari R, Collins N, et al. Primary ciliary dyskinesia: current state of the art. Arch Dis Child. 2007; 92(12):1136–1140

[13] Treacy K, Tunney M, Elborn JS, et al. Mucociliary clearance in cystic fibrosis: physiology and pharmacological treatments. Paediatr Child Health. 2011; 21(9):425–430

[14] Benninger MS, Stokken, Janalee K. Acute rhinosinusitis: pathogenesis, treatment, and complications. Cummings Otolaryngology 2015 Jan 2:724–730.e2

[15] Heikkinen T, Järvinen A. The common cold. Lancet. 2003; 361(9351): 51–59

[16] Fokkens WJ, Lund VJ, Mullol J, et al. EPOS 2012: European position paper on rhinosinusitis and nasal polyps 2012. A summary for otorhinolaryngologists. Rhinology. 2012; 50(1):1–12

[17] Benninger M, Brook I, Farrell DJ. Disease severity in acute bacterial rhinosinusitis is greater in patients infected with Streptococcus pneumoniae than in those infected with Haemophilus influenzae. Otolaryngol Head Neck Surg. 2006; 135(4):523–528

[18] Brook I, Gober AE. Frequency of recovery of pathogens from the nasopharynx of children with acute maxillary sinusitis before and after the introduction of vaccination with the 7-valent pneumococcal vaccine. Int J Pediatr Otorhinolaryngol. 2007; 71(4):575–579

[19] Payne SC, Benninger MS. Staphylococcus aureus is a major pathogen in acute bacterial rhinosinusitis: a meta-analysis. Clin Infect Dis. 2007; 45(10):e121–e127

[20] Hermens WA, Merkus FW. The influence of drugs on nasal ciliary movement. Pharm Res. 1987; 4(6):445–449

[21] Behr J, Nowak D. Tobacco smoke and respiratory disease. WORLD. 2002; 58(44):9

[22] Hilberg O, Jackson AC, Swift DL, Pedersen OF. Acoustic rhinometry: evaluation of nasal cavity geometry by acoustic reflection. J Appl Physiol (1985). 1989; 66(1):295–303

[23] Cakmak O, Coşkun M, Celik H, Büyüklü F, Ozlüoğlu LN. Value of acoustic rhinometry for measuring nasal valve area. Laryngoscope. 2003; 113(2):295–302

[24] Andersen I, Camner P, Jensen PL, Philipson K, Proctor DF. A comparison of nasal and tracheobronchial clearance. Arch Environ Health. 1974; 29(5):290–293

[25] Andersen I, Proctor DF. Measurement of nasal mucociliary clearance. Eur J Respir Dis Suppl. 1983; 127:37–40

[26] De Boeck K, Proesmans M, Mortelmans L, Van Billoen B, Willems T, Jorissen M. Mucociliary transport using 99mTc-albumin colloid: a reliable screening test for primary ciliary dyskinesia. Thorax. 2005; 60(5):414–417

[27] Pallanch J, Jorissen M. Objective assessment of nasal function. Cummings Otolaryngology. 4th ed. Vol. 40. 644–657

[28] Svartengren K, Wiman LG, Thyberg P, Rigler R. Laser light scattering spectroscopy: a new method to measure tracheobronchial mucociliary activity. Thorax. 1989; 44(7):539–547

Chapter 3

Nasal Septum and Nasal Wall Vascularization

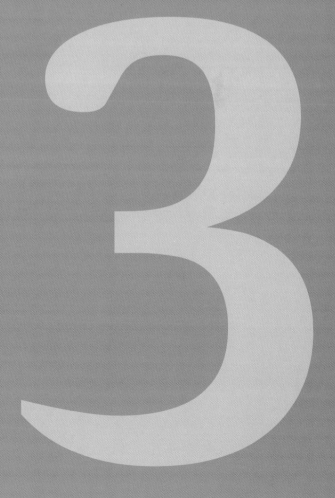

3 Nasal Septum and Nasal Wall Vascularization

Juan R. Gras-Cabrerizo, Juan Ramón Gras Albert, Elena Garcia-Garrigós, Humbert Massegur-Solench

Summary

The nasal septum and nasal wall are supplied by branches of both the external and internal carotid systems. The external carotid artery participates with the maxillary and the facial artery, whereas the internal carotid artery supplies the nasal cavity through the ethmoidal arteries originating from the ophthalmic artery.

The main branches of the maxillary artery are the sphenopalatine artery, the posterior superior alveolar artery, the infraorbital artery (IOA), the descending palatine, and the greater palatine arteries, as well as the arteries of the foramen rotundum, pterygoid canal, and pharyngeal branch (PB).

The superior labial artery (SLA) and the lateral nasal artery (LNA) arise from the facial artery and send branches to the vestibule, nasal septum, and head of the inferior turbinate.

3.1 Introduction

The nasal cavity has a rich vascular network. Arteries that supply the nasal septum and the lateral nasal wall include vessels originating from the external carotid artery (maxillary and facial artery) and from the internal carotid artery (ophthalmic artery).

3.2 Branches of Maxillary Artery (*Arteria Maxillaris*)

The maxillary artery (MA) is one of the two main end arteries from of the external carotid artery. It is located behind the neck of the mandible and passes lateral or medial to the lateral pterygoid muscle to reach the pterygopalatine fossa (PF) through the pterygopalatine fissure (pterygopalatine segment) (▸ Fig. 3.1). In the PF, the MA and its branches are located anteriorly to the neural elements. Through the PF different branches supply the orbit, the nasal cavity, the nasopharynx, the cavernous sinus, and the carotid canal. In some cases branches of the first segment of the MA (mandibular segment) can supply the nasopharynx through their extracranial branches (the middle meningeal artery and accessory meningeal artery).

3.2.1 Sphenopalatine Artery (*Arteria Sphenopalatina*)

It is the terminal branch of the MA that emerges from the superomedial part of the PF and enters the nasal cavity through the sphenopalatine foramen. This foramen is usually located in the superior meatus, although it may also be found in the middle meatus or at the transition of both meatuses, according to its location above or below the ethmoidal crest. This anatomic landmark is an optimal bone reference to localize the sphenopalatine artery because it is just posterior to this crest (▸ Fig. 3.2).

It gives off two main branches, the posterior lateral nasal artery (PLNA) and the posterior septal artery (PSA),[1,2] which can be divided into one or two trunks medial to the ethmoidal crest, before or after crossing the

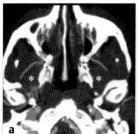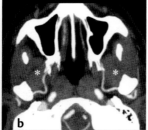

Fig. 3.1 Axial computed tomography angiography with maximum intensity projection: the maxillary artery crosses lateral (a) and medial (b) to the lateral pterygoid muscle (·).

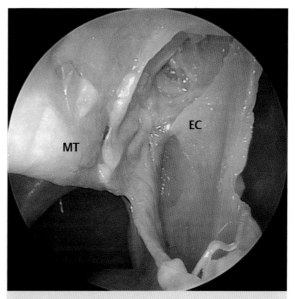

Fig. 3.2 The ethmoidal crest (EC) in the left nasal cavity. The two main branches of the sphenopalatine artery are posterior to this crest. MT, middle turbinate.

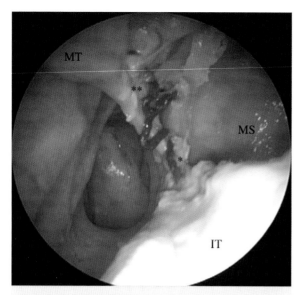

Fig. 3.3 The posterior lateral nasal artery in the left nasal cavity gives off the inferior turbinate (IT) artery (*) and middle turbinate (MT) artery (**). MS, maxillary sinus.

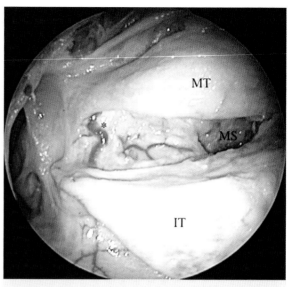

Fig. 3.4 The posterior lateral nasal artery in the left nasal cavity gives off branches to the mucosa of the fontanelle and maxillary sinus (MS) (*). IT, inferior turbinate; MT, middle turbinate.

sphenopalatine foramen. It is rarely possible to identify more than two trunks.[1,3] The PLNA supplies the region of the lateral nasal wall giving off branches to the inferior turbinate (inferior turbinate artery), middle turbinate (middle turbinate artery), mucosa of the fontanelle, and to the mucosa of the maxillary sinus[4] (▶ Fig. 3.3, ▶ Fig. 3.4). In approximately 20% of cases this artery supplies the superior turbinate.[5] The inferior turbinate artery enters a bony canal and runs anteriorly along the turbinate. It usually gives off two terminal branches, within or adjacent to the bone, supplying the mucosa of the turbinate (▶ Fig. 3.5). The artery gives off several small vessels to the maxillary sinus and to the ethmoidal complex. The middle turbinate artery gives off several branches, some of which run along the medial surface of the turbinate whereas the other branches supply the lateral turbinate surface and anterior ethmoidal complex (see ▶ Fig. 3.3).

The PSA crosses the anterior wall of the sphenoid sinus in a subperiosteal plane, between the choana and sphenoidal ostium. In most cases the artery bifurcates into the superior and inferior branches (▶ Fig. 3.6). In this area it supplies the superior turbinate (superior turbinate artery), sphenoid sinus, and posterior ethmoid complex. The superior turbinate artery can arise from the superior division of the PSA or directly from the trunk of the PSA.[6] The PSA branches on the nasal septum irrigating the inferior two-thirds. The distal extreme of the inferior branch of the PSA, the nasopalatine artery, vascularizes the inferior septal area and ends in the incisive canal where it anastomoses with the greater palatine artery (GPA).[1,2] Furthermore, the PSA presents anastomosis in the septal area with the ethmoidal arteries and with branches from the SLA (▶ Fig. 3.7).

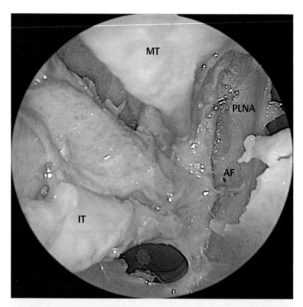

Fig. 3.5 Two terminal branches along the inferior turbinate in the left nasal cavity. AF, accessory foramen; IT, inferior turbinate; MS, maxillary sinus; MT, middle turbinate; PLNA, posterior lateral nasal artery.

3.2.2 Posterior Superior Alveolar Artery (*Arteria Alveolaris Superior Posterior*)

The posterior superior alveolar artery (PSAA) usually represents the first branch of the pterygopalatine segment of the MA. It runs close to the periosteum of the convexity

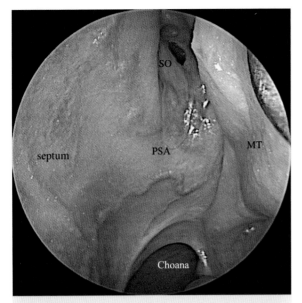

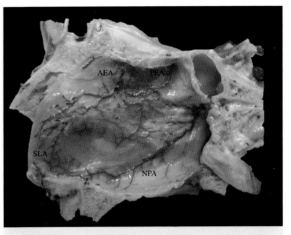

Fig. 3.7 Nasal septum vascularization. AEA, anterior ethmoidal artery; NPA, nasopalatine artery; PEA, posterior ethmoidal artery; SLA, superior labial artery.

Fig. 3.6 The posterior septal artery (PSA) crosses between the choana and the sphenoidal ostium (SO) in the left nasal cavity. The artery bifurcates into superior and inferior branches. MT, middle turbinate.

of the maxillary tuberosity and divides into two branches: a lateral descending vessel (dental branch) and an internal vessel (peridental branch). This internal branch perforates the tuberosity of the maxilla and courses endosseously supplying the mucosa of the maxillary sinus and anastomosing with the IOA[2,4,7] (▶ Fig. 3.8).

3.2.3 Infraorbital Artery (*Arteria Infraorbitalis*)

The infraorbital artery (IOA) originates from the MA or from a common trunk with the PSAA. The artery enters the maxillary sinus through the inferior orbital fissure. It runs into the infraorbital groove, which then becomes an infraorbital canal and emerges through the infraorbital foramen (see ▶ Fig. 3.8). Through a wide middle antrostomy or through an accessory ostium, we can observe the artery running anterolaterally in the roof of the maxillary sinus (▶ Fig. 3.9). Within the infraorbital canal, it gives off branches to the mucosa of the roof, the medial and anterior wall of the maxillary sinus (anterior superior alveolar arteries). At the infraorbital foramen it can anastomose with the SLA and the dorsal nasal artery (terminal branch of the ophthalmic artery).[4,7,8,9]

3.2.4 Descending Palatine Artery and the Greater Palatine Artery (*Arteria Palatine Descendens and Arteria Palatine Major*)

The descending palatine artery (DPA) originates from the deep part of the PF. It is located anterior and medial to

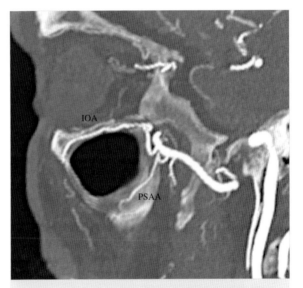

Fig. 3.8 Sagittal computed tomography angiography with maximum intensity projection. The infraorbital artery (IOA) runs along the roof of the maxillary sinus and the posterior superior alveolar artery (PSAA) courses in the lateral wall of the maxillary sinus.

the infraorbital canal and descends slightly obliquely through the greater palatine canal (▶ Fig. 3.10). In its descent route to the hard palate, it can give off some small branches. In about 5 to 13% of cases an accessory foramen can be found in the palatine bone of this canal. It is inferior to and smaller than the sphenopalatine foramen and is crossed by a small vessel from the DPA to the inferior turbinate[3,10,11] (see ▶ Fig. 3.5). Then the DPA passes through the greater palatine foramen to the posterior area of the hard palate. In this journey the artery changes its name to the greater palatine artery (GPA). It

21

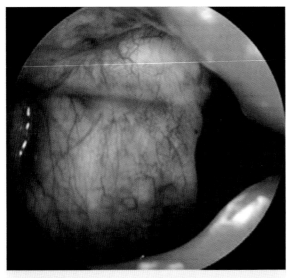

Fig. 3.9 The infraorbital canal seen through a middle meatal antrostomy.

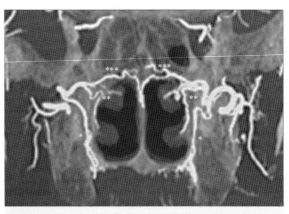

Fig. 3.10 Coronal computed tomography angiography with maximum intensity projection. The descending palatine artery (DPA) descends through the greater palatine canal (*). It can be noted the bifurcation of the sphenopalatine artery. The posterior lateral nasal artery (PLNA) (**) gives off branches to the inferior and middle turbinate and the posterior septal artery (PSA) course along the choana (***).

supplies the floor of the nasal cavity, maxillary sinus, and it anastomoses with the nasopalatine artery to supply the nasal septum.

3.2.5 Artery of Foramen Rotundum

The three posterior branches of the distal MA are, from superolateral to inferomedial, the artery of the foramen rotundum (AFR), artery of the pterygoid canal, and the pterygovaginal artery. To localize these vascular structures, we must perform a dissection posterior and superior to the sphenopalatine foramen. The AFR runs along the maxillary nerve and enters the foramen rotundum. The artery supplies the roof of the nasopharynx. It can anastomose with the inferolateral trunk of the cavernous segment of the internal carotid artery.[12]

3.2.6 Artery of Pterygoid Canal or Vidian Artery (*Arteria Canalis Pterygoidei*)

The rest of the first aortic arch is called the primitive mandibular artery or the Vidian artery (VA) in adults. It arises within the PF and passes posteriorly through the pterygoid canal to the foramen lacerum (petrous internal carotid artery) (▶ Fig. 3.11). In the 30% of cases the VA can inversely arise from the internal carotid artery to the PF.[13] It supplies the mucosa of the PF, nasopharynx, and eustachian tube. It participates in a complex vascular network anastomosing with the meningeal arteries, the ascending

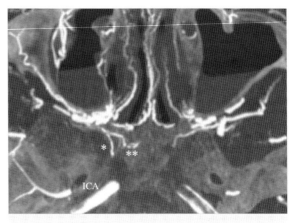

Fig. 3.11 Axial computed tomography angiography with maximum intensity projection. The vidian artery (*) passes through the pterygoid canal, from the pterygopalatine fossa to the petrous internal carotid artery (ICA). The pharyngeal branch (**) courses the roof of the nasopharynx.

and descending palatine arteries, and the ascending pharyngeal artery.[12,13]

3.2.7 Pharyngeal Branch or Pterygovaginal Artery (*Ramus Pharyngeus*)

The pharyngeal branch (PB) originates close to the VA or forms a common trunk with it. Then it passes through the palatovaginal canal and supplies the posterior aspect of the roof of the nasopharynx, posterior portion of the

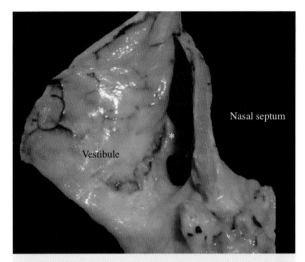

Fig. 3.12 Right nasal vestibule. Branches from the lateral nasal artery (LNA) and superior labial artery (SLA) supplying the nasal vestibule and the head of the inferior turbinate (*).

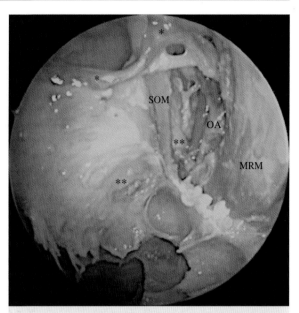

Fig. 3.13 Intraorbital origin of the ethmoidal arteries in the left nasal cavity. Anterior ethmoidal route (*). Posterior ethmoidal route (**). MRM, medial rectus muscle; OA, ophthalmic artery; SOM, superior oblique muscle.

choana, sphenoidal sinus, and eustachian tube (see ► Fig. 3.11). In some cases the artery arises directly from the PSA and not from the MA. There may be an anastomotic artery between the MA and ascending pharyngeal artery or ascending palatine artery.[6,14]

3.3 Branches of Facial Artery (*Arteria Facialis*)

3.3.1 Superior Labial Artery (*Arteria Labialis Superior*)

The superior labial artery (SLA) originates from the facial artery near the lateral end of the oral fissure. It passes between the orbicularis oris muscle and mucosa, vascularizing the lip. Septal branches ascend vertically and supply the columella, membranous septum, and anterior area(s) of the septum (see ► Fig. 3.7). In approximately half of the cases, it runs as a single trunk and as ramified branches in the other cases.[2,15] Between 1 and 7% of cases the SLA is absent and the facial artery terminates as a rudimentary branch.[16,17]

3.3.2 Lateral Nasal Artery (*Arteria Lateralis Nasi*)

The lateral nasal artery (LNA) can arise from the SLA or directly from the facial artery. It is the main supplying artery of the alar area, nasal tip, and nasal vestibule.[15] Some branches from the SLA or LNA can not only vascularize the nasal vestibule and nasal septum but also reach the head of the inferior turbinate (► Fig. 3.12).

3.4 Branches of Ophthalmic Artery (*Arteria Ophthalmica*)

The ethmoidal arteries (*arteria ethmoidalis anterior* and *arteria ethmoidalis posterior*) arise from the ophthalmic artery in its intraorbital route. The anterior ethmoidal artery (AEA) passes through the superior oblique muscle and medial rectus muscle, describing a curvature before being placed on the ethmoidal roof. The posterior ethmoidal artery (PEA) runs superior to the superior oblique muscle (► Fig. 3.13). Between 14 and 16% of the cases the PEA can originate from a common trunk with the supraorbital artery.[18] Both ethmoidal arteries reach the roof of the ethmoidal complex through the ethmoidal foramina going through the lamina papyracea. AEA and PEA run along the ethmoidal roof from lateral to medial, reaching the lateral lamella of the cribriform plate (► Fig. 3.14). Depending on the pneumatization of the ethmoidal roof, the ethmoidal arteries may be more or less evident. The bulging of the artery canal is usually more evident for the AEA than for the posterior canal. The AEA describes an oblique route allowing identifying a beak in the lamina papyracea. The mean length of the anterior ethmoidal canal is about 8.5 mm with an angle of 37 degrees in the skull base.[19] In some cases the AEA can present a mesentery suspended from the skull base and it is possible to be dehiscent inferiorly. The posterior ethmoidal canal is usually embedded in the skull base and consequently less

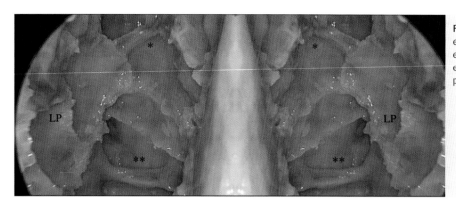

Fig. 3.14 Bilateral roof of the ethmoidal complex. Anterior ethmoidal canal (*). Posterior ethmoidal canal (**). LP, lamina papyracea.

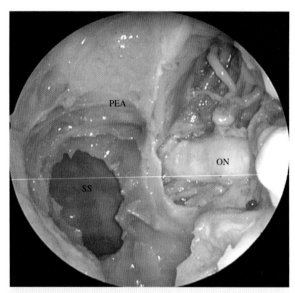

Fig. 3.15 Relationship between left posterior ethmoidal artery (PEA) and optic nerve (ON). The inferior and the middle rectus muscles have been removed. SS, sphenoidal sinus.

identifiable. The mean length of the posterior ethmoidal canal is about 7.1 mm with an angle of approximately 7.1 degrees in the skull base.[19] The most superior part of the basal lamella of the ethmoidal bulla is the landmark to find the AEA. In most cases the AEA is located behind this wall. The PEA crosses the ethmoid roof through a canal anterior to the superior attachment of the anterior wall of the sphenoid sinus. The mean distance in between the AEA and PEA is about 10 to 12 mm, and it is important for surgical approaches to consider the proximity of the PEA with the optic nerve, around 4 to 7 mm posteriorly[1,19] (▶ Fig. 3.15). The AEA gives off the anterior meningeal artery that enters intracranial below the dura mater and descends through the cribriform plate, supplying the anterior superior part of the septum (anterior septal branches) and anterior ethmoidal cells, frontal sinus, and middle turbinate (anterior lateral nasal branches)[2] (see ▶ Fig. 3.7).

The AEA can be absent unilaterally in 7 to 14% of cases and in 2% bilaterally. In these cases a branch from the PEA[20,21] supplies the vascularization. The PEA supplies the dura mater above the cribriform plate with a meningeal branch, and the posterior ethmoidal cells, superior turbinate, and posterior superior area of the nasal septum with nasal branches. Between 25 and 42% of cases it is possible to find a middle ethmoidal artery (MEA), and in 14% the MEA can be bilateral. It seems to be smaller and thinner than the AEA and is located between both the ethmoidal arteries, usually closer to the PEA.[22]

The venous system is more variable and complex than the arterial system. The venous drainage generally runs parallel to the arterial supply. Veins that go along with the branches originate from the MA, in the infratemporal and PF, drain mainly into the pterygoid plexus. In addition, the inferior ophthalmic vein from the inferior palpebral and lacrimal gland can drain through the inferior orbital fissure into the pterygoid plexus.[9] The pterygoid plexus connects posteriorly with the maxillary vein, which anastomoses with the retromandibular vein. Anteriorly, the plexus communicates with the facial vein on the face. Therefore, some emissary veins connect this plexus with the cavernous sinuses through little emissary foramina.[2,9] The ethmoidal and lacrimal veins drain into the superior ophthalmic vein (SOV), which drains in the cavernous sinus through the superior orbital fissure. The nasofrontal vein drains in the angular vein and is related to the SOV.

References

[1] Lund VJ, Stammberger H, Fokkens WJ, et al. European position paper on the anatomical terminology of the internal nose and paranasal sinuses. Rhinol Suppl. 2014(24):1–34

[2] Dauber W, ed. Feneis: Nomenclatura anatómica ilustrada. 5th ed. Barcelona, Spain: Elsevier Masson; 2007

[3] Gras-Cabrerizo JR, Ademá-Alcover JM, Gras-Albert JR, et al. Anatomical and surgical study of the sphenopalatine artery branches. Eur Arch Otorhinolaryngol. 2014; 271(7):1947–1951

[4] Rosano G, Taschieri S, Gaudy JF, Del Fabbro M. Maxillary sinus vascularization: a cadaveric study. J Craniofac Surg. 2009; 20(3):940–943

[5] Lee HY, Kim HU, Kim SS, et al. Surgical anatomy of the sphenopalatine artery in lateral nasal wall. Laryngoscope. 2002; 112(10):1813–1818

[6] Zhang X, Wang EW, Wei H, et al. Anatomy of the posterior septal artery with surgical implications on the vascularized pedicled naso-septal flap. Head Neck. 2014

[7] Solar P, Geyerhofer U, Traxler H, Windisch A, Ulm C, Watzek G. Blood supply to the maxillary sinus relevant to sinus floor elevation proce-dures. Clin Oral Implants Res. 1999; 10(1):34–44

[8] Hayreh SS. Orbital vascular anatomy. Eye (Lond). 2006; 20(10):1130–1144

[9] Drake L, Gray H. Gray's Atlas of Anatomy. 1st ed. Philadelphia, PA: Churchill Livingstone; 2008

[10] Wareing MJ, Padgham ND. Osteologic classification of the sphenopa-latine foramen. Laryngoscope. 1998; 108(1 Pt 1):125–127

[11] Padgham N, Vaughan-Jones R. Cadaver studies of the anatomy of arterial supply to the inferior turbinates. J R Soc Med. 1991; 84(12):728–730

[12] Tanoue S, Kiyosue H, Mori H, Hori Y, Okahara M, Sagara Y. Maxillary artery: functional and imaging anatomy for safe and effective trans-catheter treatment. Radiographics. 2013; 33(7):e209–e224

[13] Osborn AG. The Vidian artery: normal and pathologic anatomy. Radi-ology. 1980; 136(2):373–378

[14] Karligkiotis A, Volpi L, Abbate V, et al. Palatovaginal (pharyngeal) artery: clinical implication and surgical experience. Eur Arch Otorhi-nolaryngol. 2014; 271(10):2839–2843

[15] Pinar YA, Bilge O, Govsa F. Anatomic study of the blood supply of perioral region. Clin Anat. 2005; 18(5):330–339

[16] Loukas M, Hullett J, Louis RG, Jr, et al. A detailed observation of varia-tions of the facial artery, with emphasis on the superior labial artery. Surg Radiol Anat. 2006; 28(3):316–324

[17] Lee SH, Gil YC, Choi YJ, Tansatit T, Kim HJ, Hu KS. Topographic anat-omy of the superior labial artery for dermal filler injection. Plast Reconstr Surg. 2015; 135(2):445–450

[18] Erdogmus S, Govsa F. Accurate course and relationships of the intra-orbital part of the ophthalmic artery in the sagittal plane. Minim Invasive Neurosurg. 2007; 50(4):202–208

[19] Monjas-Cánovas I, García-Garrigós E, Arenas-Jiménez JJ, Abarca-Oli-vas J, Sánchez-Del Campo F, Gras-Albert JR. [Radiological anatomy of the ethmoidal arteries: CT cadaver study]. Acta Otorrinolaringol Esp. 2011; 62(5):367–374

[20] Lang J, Schäfer K. [Ethmoidal arteries: origin, course, regions supplied and anastomoses]. Acta Anat (Basel). 1979; 104(2):183–197

[21] Yang YX, Lu QK, Liao JC, Dang RS. Morphological characteristics of the anterior ethmoidal artery in ethmoid roof and endoscopic localiza-tion. Skull Base. 2009; 19(5):311–317

[22] Wang L, Youseef A, Al Qahtani AA, et al. Endoscopic anatomy of the middle ethmoidal artery. Int Forum Allergy Rhinol. 2014; 4(2):164–168

Chapter 4
Nasal Perforation Etiology

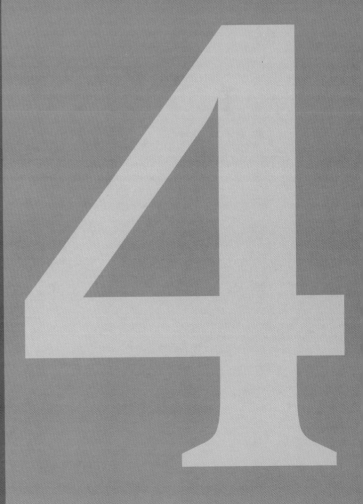

4 Nasal Perforation Etiology

Mauricio López-Chacón, Arturo Cordero Castillo, Cristobal Langdon, Francesca Jaume, Isam Alobid

Summary

The etiology of nasal septal perforation (NSP) is very variable; the most common cause is traumatic postsurgical procedure. However, the presence of an NSP could also be the first clinical manifestation of a systemic inflammatory disease such as granulomatous polyangiitis, sarcoidosis, lupus erythematosus, neoplasia, or infection. An adequate medical history and physical examination are the most relevant tools when establishing the differential diagnosis. Complementary tests that can also aid in the diagnosis include laboratory tests (complete blood cell count [CBC], specific antibodies), imaging tests (computed tomographic [CT] scans), or biopsies.

4.1 Introduction

Nasal septal perforation (NSP) is defined as a communication between the two nasal cavities secondary to a defect in any portion of the mucosa, submucosa, and the perichondrium, as well as in the osteocartilage septum (▶ Fig. 4.1). NSP can have an iatrogenic or pathological origin.[1,2]

Previous studies report that the approximate prevalence of NSP in the general population is 1%, although its exact prevalence is difficult to determine.[3,4] Between 15 and 39% of patients with NSP do not experience any symptoms and are diagnosed during a routine ENT (ear-nose-throat) examination.[1,5] The localization and the size

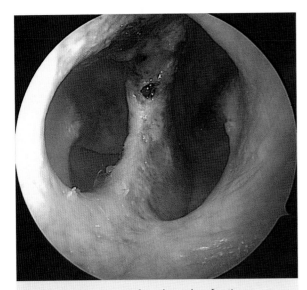

Fig. 4.1 Endoscopic view of nasal septal perforation.

of the perforation can influence in the presence of symptomatology.[1]

Regarding the localization of the nasal perforations, 92% are located in the anterior portion of the septum and 8% are either posterior or superior.[4] Anterior perforations are more frequently caused by trauma and are usually associated with more symptomatology, whereas posterior or superior perforations are mostly associated with systemic diseases.

The most frequent symptoms associated with NSP include epistaxis (58%), crusting (43%), obstruction (39%), pain (17%), and whistling (15%).[1,4]

The etiology of NSP is very variable. The most common are traumatic secondary to bilateral laceration of the septal mucosa during septoplasty.[2,5,6] However, the presence of an NSP could also be the first clinical manifestation of a systemic inflammatory disease such as granulomatous polyangiitis, sarcoidosis, lupus erythematosus, neoplasia, or infeccions.[3,6,7,8] Nowadays there has been an increase in NSP prevalence secondary to the consumption of licit and illicit intranasal drugs.[3]

The authors discuss the pathogenesis and principal causes of NSP, including traumatic, nasal drug use, occupational exposure, and neoplasia. Systemic causes are discussed in greater detail in Chapter 5.

4.2 Pathogenesis

The nasal septal mucoperichondrium is in charge of providing blood supply to the quadrangular cartilage. NSP usually occurs when there has been an interruption in the vascular supply in both sides of the septal mucosa at almost the same location.[1,4,5,8]

Four stages have been described in the development of NSP. The first stage consists in mucosal irritation accompanied with rhinorrhea. During the second stage, a blanching occurs at the anterior-inferior portion of the septal mucosa at the Kiesselbach area, which has less vascularization and increased adherence to the cartilage. This inflammatory process leads to the production of crusting and nasal picking, which increases the risk of infection in the affected area. During these initial steps there is also a loss of the mucosal and submucosal layer, without affecting the perichondrial layer. If the mucosal layer does not regenerate adequately, a loss of the perichondrial layer occurs followed by ulceration and necrosis of the septal cartilage. The borders of the perforation are covered with atrophic epithelium that is more susceptible to bleeding and crust formation. This is also affected by the change in airflow. If no other insults occur, the border cicatrization is produced in approximately 3 months.[1,4,5,8]

4.3 Etiology

In the following paragraphs the different local etiologies associated with NSP are discussed in greater detail. As shown in ▶ Table 4.1, the etiologies can be grouped in traumatic, intranasal drugs use and neoplasms. Systemic diseases (inflammatory and infectious) are discussed in Chapter 5.

4.3.1 Traumatic Causes

Some studies report that the prevalence of traumatic NSP is around 39% of the total amount of NSP.[5] Self-inflicted trauma, accidental trauma, or medical procedure-related trauma are the most common causes.[5]

Approximately 1 to 8% of nasal septoplasties are complicated with NSP.[9] It should be highlighted that a higher percentage (~17%) has been reported with submucosal nasal septum resection technique.[6]

Studies performed in cadavers have determined that the major mechanical tensile strength of the septal lining is localized in the perichondrial layer. Therefore, a correct dissection of the subperichondrial plane during septal surgery provides a stronger septal flap and may prevent the development of NSP during nasal surgery.[10]

Other important factors that should be taken into account during a septoplasty is the precarious irrigation of the quadrangular cartilage, because the risk of NSP increases if the blood supply is disrupted on both sides of the mucosa in approximately the same area.[1]

Allergic rhinitis (AR) has also been associated with an increased risk of NSP following septoplasty due to the mucosal epithelial damage during the allergic season. However, this has not been proven when comparing the incidence of NSP after septoplasty between patients with and without AR.[11]

Different suture techniques have been developed to prevent postsurgical complication after nasal packing and nasal splints.[12] Many studies have concluded that the risk of synechiae, and hematomas are lower when using nasal splints and suturing compared with nasal packings.[12] However, those studies have not found significant differences when comparing the use of nasal packing, haemostatic suturing techniques, and nasal splints to prevent the formation of NSP or infections.[9,12]

4.3.2 Intranasal Drug Abuse

The use of illicit drugs, in particular cocaine, has been highly associated with NSP. Although licit drugs, including vasoconstrictors and intranasal steroids, have also been related with NSP, their incidence is quite lower.[6]

Cocaine

Cocaine is one of the most trafficked illicit drugs worldwide. In the 1980s approximately 22 million of Americans used illicit cocaine whereas 4 million were using cocaine at least once in a month. Nowadays the frequency has decreased to 4 million, with an at least once-a-month use in 1.3 million and once-a-week use in 64,000 individuals.[13] The incidence of NSP in cocaine consumers is 4.8%.[1]

Owebs reported the first case of NSP secondary to cocaine consumption in 1912.[13] The chronic consumption of cocaine can cause a variety of intranasal destructive lesions, including NSP, lateral nasal wall and/or hard palate destruction, etc. It can also cause manifestations that can mimic multisystemic diseases presenting with mild facial destructive lesion associated with a positive antineutrophil cytoplasmic antibodies (ANCA) and histopathologic alterations, which causes difficulty in distinguishing it between granulomatosis with polyangiitis (GPA), neoplasms, autoimmune diseases, or infections.

The common pathophysiology shared by patients using these types of drugs is the ischemia and the chemical irritation. The ischemia will cause a necrosis of the mucosa and septal cartilage secondary to the inhibition of noradrenaline reuptake.[1] This ischemia is often aggravated

Table 4.1 Causes of nasal septal ulcerations (modified from[4,8])

Nasal septal perforation	
Traumatic/iatrogenic	Septal surgery
	Chemical cautery
	Nasal packing
	Nasogastric probe
	Nasal fracture
	Foreign body
	Self-inflicted
Nasal drug abuse	Decongestant
	Corticoids
	Cocaine
Occupational exposure	Chemical irritants
	Physical irritants
	Heavy metal
Inflammatory	Wegener's granulomatosis
	Sarcoidosis
	Systemic lupus erythematosus
	Rheumatoid arthritis
	Crohn's disease
	Dermatomyositis
	Sarcoidosis
Infectious	Syphilis
	HIV
	Fungal infections
	Leprosy
	Tuberculosis
Neoplasms	Non-Hodgkin lymphoma
	Squamous cell carcinoma
	Adenoid cystic carcinoma
	Basal cell carcinoma
	Esthesioneuroblastoma
	Rhabdomyosarcoma

Abbreviation: HIV, human immunodeficiency virus.

with the use of intranasal vasoconstrictors to prevent the associated rebound hyperemia.[14]

The chemical irritation is related to the excipients that are mixed with cocaine, such as dextrose, lactose, mannitol, talc, borax caffeine amphetamines, and heroin.[13,14] The mucosal lesions caused by the excipients are aggravated by local trauma when cocaine abusers pick their nose with an instrument like a pen or pencil to relief discomfort, which can in turn cause infections. The type and extension of infections vary between cocaine abusers due to different hygienic habits and antibiotic use.[14]

The pathogenesis of the systemic effects of cocaine is poorly understood and it could possibly be associated with predisposing factors as well as inflammatory, infectious, proapoptotic, and autoimmune factors.[13,14] It has been hypothesized that one of the possible mechanisms that could explain the extension of the intranasal destruction could be related to the destructive effects of cocaine by increasing cellular apoptosis.[13,14] This could also be influenced by the time of exposure and dosage.[13,14]

It is difficult to diagnose it due to the low incidence of this disease. Its principal differential diagnosis is GPA.[14] There are patients with systemic effects who do not present intranasal lesions with concrete histopathologic findings. However, the absence of stromal granulomas with giant cells, microabscesses, and deeply located necrosis characteristic of GPA help point toward the diagnosis.

For an adequate approach to these type of patients, obtaining a complete medical history with toxicologic tests, TUNEL (terminal deoxynucleotidyl transferase dUTP nick end labeling) assay, and magnetic resonance imaging (MRI) is recommended. The presence of HNE-ANCA–positive antibodies is of great aid in the diagnosis.

Intranasal Vasoconstrictors

The use of topical vasoconstrictors has always been associated with NSP. However, this association has been poorly supported by the literature.

Studies performed in rats have shown that an exposure with topical vasoconstrictors (oxymetazoline) for 15 days at dose 10 to 30 times more than the recommended have been associated with an increased incidence in NSP.[15] Another study, also performed in rats, showed that the use of oxymetazoline in nasal mucosa increased ischemic changes, congestion, arterial thrombosis, and necrosis.[16] Although, these results have not been confirmed in human studies, surveillance reports of the Food and Drug Administration (FDA) from 1997 through 2007 report two cases of NSP associated with the administration of oxymetazoline.[1] However, in the United States 150 million mL of oxymetazoline were sold during 2006 and there were no cases of NSP reported.[1] Therefore, it seems that oxymetazoline mechanism of action might cause NSP at very high doses, but in human there might be other factors involved that could influence its development.

Intranasal Steroids

The first intranasal topical steroid used was dexamethasone in 1965 and since then there has been an increase in the medical indications, as well as the active substances that have been used as intranasal steroids have been changing.[1] Nowadays intranasal steroids are used at higher doses and for longer times, which explains why there are numerous studies focused on its adverse effects. One of the described adverse effects is NSP. Initially it was found in studies performed in rats that excipients, for instance benzalkonium chloride, were associated with mucosal irritation.[17] However, there has been conflictive evidence in humans of delayed or contact sensitivity of intranasal topic steroids. It has been hypothesized that the association could be secondary to vasoconstrictive effects of intranasal topical steroids. However, a study with laser Doppler flowmetry did not detect changes in vascular irrigation after the administration of budesonide.[18] Although association studies have found a relation between intranasal topic steroids and allergic dermatitis,[19] clinical studies have not been able to replicate this association.[20] Nevertheless, the FDA has catalogued the association between intranasal steroids and NSP as rare or not clearly defined incidence rate association.[1] A prevalence study performed in Sweden described NSP as an uncommon side effect with an incidence of less than 1/1,000.[21] Because topical intranasal steroids are widely used, the ENT strongly recommends a complete nasal examination to discard mucosal alterations.

4.3.3 Occupational Exposure

NSP of occupational origin is frequently underestimated.[22] Most cases reported in the literature are associated with the occupational exposure of corrosive chemicals.[23] A *corrosive chemical* is defined as a product that is capable of causing an irreversible destruction or alteration of live tissue, due to a chemical reaction on the contact site.[24] Even though there is a long list of corrosive agents, the scientific evidence linking them with NSP is low.[23]

There are cases of NSP in workers that have been exposed to nickel, copper, arsenic, aluminum, and chrome.[23,25] The exposure to chromic acid mist in electroplating industry workers is the best studied example of NSP secondary to corrosive chemical exposure.[22,23,25] The prevalence of NSP in workers exposed to chromic acid mist lies between 20 and 30%. Patients usually present with nasal obstruction, sneezing, and itching like any other rhinitis, but they also report an increase in the incidence of symptoms such as dryness, epistaxis, and formation of crust.[26] The time of exposure for these symptoms to appear varies between 6 and 12 months, depending on the intensity of exposure, although it could also occur after a few weeks of exposure.[23] Early-onset cases seem to be related to low hygiene standards and nose picking with contaminated fingers.[22]

Preventive measures include the use of dusk masks, hand washing at the end of the work shift, regular cleaning of the floors, and proper exhaust ventilation.[25] It has also been shown that the use of ethylenediaminetetraacetic acid (EDTA) ointment with 10% $CaNO_3$ applied regularly over the mucosa could help avoid the formation of NSP in workers exposed to chrome. This ointment reduces the hexavalent form of chrome to a trivalent form that is less irritant and corrosive.[26]

Otorhinolaryngologists should search for antecedents of exposure to corrosives chemicals at the workplace when evaluating a patient with NSP.

4.3.4 Neoplasm

Different neoplasms are associated with NSP (see ▶ Table 4.1). The lethal midline granuloma–nasal natural killer (LMG-NK) cell lymphoma is a very rare entity, with a male predominance and a wide-age range.[4] This lesion is characterized by an unilateral ulcerative process with cartilage loss, friable mucosa, crusting, and loss of nasal structure often extended toward the palate, maxillary sinus, and upper lip.[4] Treatment involves radiotherapy and the survival rate at 5 years is 20%.[4]

The main location of squamous cell carcinomas, adenoid cystic carcinomas, and melanomas are not usually the midline, but it should be ruled out in the differential diagnosis.[27] Tissue biopsy is fundamental tool in the differential diagnosis of neoplasms.[5] Although neoplasms in the nasal septum are extremely rare causes of NSP, they should be discarded when evaluating a patient.

4.3.5 Systemic Diseases

Systemic diseases are discussed in greater detail in Chapter 5.

4.4 Conclusion

As it has been described, there are many etiologies associated with NSP, and establishing the diagnosis is a challenge for the physician. An adequate medical history and physical examination are the most relevant tools when establishing the differential diagnosis. Complementary tests that can also aid information in the diagnosis include laboratory tests (CBC, specific antibodies), imaging tests (CT scans), or biopsies. With regards to the biopsy, in the past it was considered a fundamental test when assessing nasal septum pathology. However, recent studies have shown that its use is most relevant when there is a clinical suspicion of malignancy.

References

[1] Lanier B, Kai G, Marple B, Wall GM. Pathophysiology and progression of nasal septal perforation. Ann Allergy Asthma Immunol. 2007; 99 (6):473–479, quiz 480–481, 521

[2] Moon IJ, Kim S-W, Han DH, et al. Predictive factors for the outcome of nasal septal perforation repair. Auris Nasus Larynx. 2011; 38(1): 52–57

[3] Oberg D, Akerlund A, Johansson L, Bende M. Prevalence of nasal septal perforation: the Skövde population-based study. Rhinology. 2003; 41(2):72–75

[4] Sardana K, Goel K. Nasal septal ulceration. Clin Dermatol. 2014; 32 (6):817–826

[5] Diamantopoulos II, Jones NS. The investigation of nasal septal perforations and ulcers. J Laryngol Otol. 2001; 115(7):541–544

[6] Døsen LK, Haye R, Døsen LK. Nasal septal perforation 1981–2005: changes in etiology, gender and size. BMC Ear Nose Throat Disord. 2007; 7:1

[7] Alobid I, Guilemany JM, Mullol J. Nasal manifestations of systemic illnesses. Curr Allergy Asthma Rep. 2004; 4(3):208–216

[8] Fornazieri MA, Moreira JH, Pilan R, Voegels RL. Perfuração do septo nasal: etiologia e diagnóstico perforation of nasal septum: etiology and diagnosis. Arq Int Otorrinolaringol. 2010; 14(4):467–471

[9] Rettinger G, Kirsche H. Complications in septoplasty. Facial Plast Surg. 2006; 22(4):289–297

[10] Kim DW, Egan KK, O'Grady K, Toriumi DM. Biomechanical strength of human nasal septal lining: comparison of the constituent layers. Laryngoscope. 2005; 115(8):1451–1453

[11] Topal O, Celik SB, Erbek S, Erbek SS. Risk of nasal septal perforation following septoplasty in patients with allergic rhinitis. Eur Arch Otorhinolaryngol. 2011; 268(2):231–233

[12] Deniz M, Ciftçi Z, Işık A, Demirel OB, Gültekin E. The impact of different nasal packings on postoperative complications. Am J Otolaryngol. 2014; 35(5):554–557

[13] Smith JC, Kacker A, Anand VK. Midline nasal and hard palate destruction in cocaine abusers and cocaine's role in rhinologic practice. Ear Nose Throat J. 2002; 81(3):172–177

[14] Trimarchi M, Bertazzoni G, Bussi M. Cocaine induced midline destructive lesions. Rhinology. 2014; 52(2):104–111

[15] DeBernardis JF, Winn M, Kerkman DJ, Kyncl JJ, Buckner S, Horrom B. A new nasal decongestant, A-57219: a comparison with oxymetazoline. J Pharm Pharmacol. 1987; 39(9):760–763

[16] Dokuyucu R, Gokce H, Sahan M, et al. Systemic side effects of locally used oxymetazoline. Int J Clin Exp Med. 2015; 8(2):2674–2678

[17] Berg OH, Lie K, Steinsvåg SK. The effects of topical nasal steroids on rat respiratory mucosa in vivo, with special reference to benzalkonium chloride. Allergy. 1997; 52(6):627–632

[18] Cervin A, Akerlund A, Greiff L, Andersson M. The effect of intranasal budesonide spray on mucosal blood flow measured with laser Doppler flowmetry. Rhinology. 2001; 39(1):13–16

[19] Isaksson M, Bruze M, Wihl JA. Contact allergy to budesonide and perforation of the nasal septum. Contact Dermat. 1997; 37(3):133

[20] Cervin A, Hansson C, Greiff L, Andersson M. Nasal septal perforations during treatment with topical nasal glucocorticosteroids are generally not associated with contact allergy to steroids. ORL J Otorhinolaryngol Relat Spec. 2003; 65(2):103–105

[21] Cervin A, Andersson M. Intranasal steroids and septum perforation—an overlooked complication? A description of the course of events and a discussion of the causes. Rhinology. 1998; 36(3):128–132

[22] Williams N. What are the causes of a perforated nasal septum? Occup Med (Lond). 2000; 50(2):135–136

[23] Castano R, Thériault G, Gautrin D. Categorizing nasal septal perforations of occupational origin as cases of corrosive rhinitis. Am J Ind Med. 2007; 50(2):150–153

[24] Tovar R, Leikin JB. Irritants and corrosives. Emerg Med Clin North Am. 2015; 33(1):117–131

[25] Naik SM, Naik MS. Nasal septal perforations—an occupational hazard in chrome industry workers. IJPMR 2013;1:13–15

[26] Moscato G, Vandenplas O, Van Wijk RG, et al. EAACI position paper on occupational rhinitis. Respir Res 2009;10:16

[27] DiLeo MD, Miller RH, Rice JC, Butcher RB. Nasal septal squamous cell carcinoma: a chart review and meta-analysis. Laryngoscope. 1996; 106(10):1218–1222

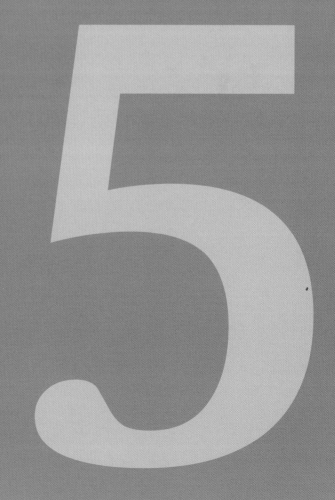

Chapter 5

Systemic Diseases Associated with Septal Perforation

5 Systemic Diseases Associated with Septal Perforation

Mauricio López-Chacón, Arturo Cordero Castillo, Cristobal Langdon, Alfonso Santamaría, Isam Alobid

Summary

Systemic and infectious diseases can present with nasal septum perforations (NSPs) either at the beginning of the symptomatology or along the evolution of the clinical manifestations. A meticulous medical history and a physical examination are essential for the diagnosis in these patients. Complementary testing, including laboratory, imaging, and biopsies, also has a relevant role in this pathology involving very distinct etiologies. Infectious diseases and multisystemic disorders (vasculitis and autoimmune diseases) are discussed in this chapter (▶ Fig. 5.1).

5.1 Infectious Diseases

Even though NSP is a rare manifestation of systemic or infectious diseases, multiple diseases have been related with septum perforations. It is very difficult to estimate the frequency of NSPs due to lack of information. In the following paragraphs the most frequent associated infections are described.

5.1.1 Tuberculosis

Approximately 260,000 of tuberculosis (TB) were reported between 2000 and 2011 in the United States and the United Kingdom.[1] The incidence of TB declined during these years in the United States (from 5.8 to 3.4 cases per 100,000), whereas the incidence increased in the United Kingdom (from 11.4 to 14.4 cases per 100,000).[1] The incidence of TB in Spain has been reported to be 13 cases per 100,000 habitants.[2,3,4]

Mycobacterium tuberculosis is the main infectious agent causing TB. There are other atypical mycobacteria such as *Mycobacterium kansasii* that can also cause similar clinical and pathologic manifestations.[5] The nasal symptoms in patients diagnosed with TB are similar to a cold with rhinorrhea and nasal obstruction.[6] The most frequent affected location is the nasopharynx, characterized by adenoid hypertrophy, rhinorrhea, and cervical lymphadenopathies. If nasal polyps are observed, they usually grow predominantly from the inferior turbinate.[5]

Primary nasal TB is a very rare finding. Butt revised the cases published during the 20th century and found 35 cases of nasal TB, of which only 12 were primary nasal TB.[7] It is rare for *M. tuberculosis* to infect the nasal mucosa nasal, because of its bactericide secretions, cilia movement, and the presence of nasal vibrissae. The main cause could be related to the inhalation of infected particles by a damaged or atrophic mucosa or by direct traumatic digital inoculation.[8] In the case of primary nasal TB, the symptomatology is usually unilateral and consists of nasal obstruction, rhinorrhea, and nosebleed when destructive lesions are present (ulcers or perforations). The most frequent location is the septum, followed by the lateral wall.[6]

The differential diagnoses include malignancy processes; inflammatory granulomatosis (Wegener's granulomatosis, sarcoidosis, leprosy, or syphilis); and viral, parasitic, or fungal infections.

The nonspecific nature of the symptoms and rareness of a nasal location usually lead to a delay in diagnosis. Although several imaging tests (computed tomography [CT], magnetic resonance imaging [MRI], and positron emission tomography–computed tomography [PET-CT]) can help delimitate the extension of the lesions, they lack diagnostic specificity.

The diagnosis should include acid-fast smear, culture, and tuberculin skin testing. With the use of polymerase chain reaction (PCR) and Xpert MTB/RIF assays for rapid diagnosis and detection of TB, treatment can be initiated earlier.[9] However, it is also important to have the biopsy samples for pathologic study and microbiologic culture, even though the results of the microbiologic culture are negative in up to 50 to 75% of cases.[5] Once the diagnosis of TB has been confirmed, the presence of pulmonary and systemic TB must be ruled out.[5,6,8]

Treatment consists of anti-TB drugs, which achieve a rapid and complete response in the majority of cases. In a series of 50 cases with nasopharynx TB, all patients were disease-free 2 years after completing the treatment.[10]

5.1.2 Leprosy

Leprosy is a potentially disabling disease causing deformities and physical disability due to an infectious agent.[6] In 2000 leprosy was eliminated, defined as a decrease in disease prevalence of less than 1 case per 10,000 habitants.[11] The prevalence and incidence of leprosy have remained constant since 2005, despite the existence of effective multidrug treatment.[12]

Leprosy is caused by *Mycobacterium leprae* and is characterized by skin and peripheral nerve damage. In advanced cases it can affect the great majority of organs, including the ears, nose, and throat.[6] The nasal mucosa is affected in 95% of patients with lepromatous leprosy and

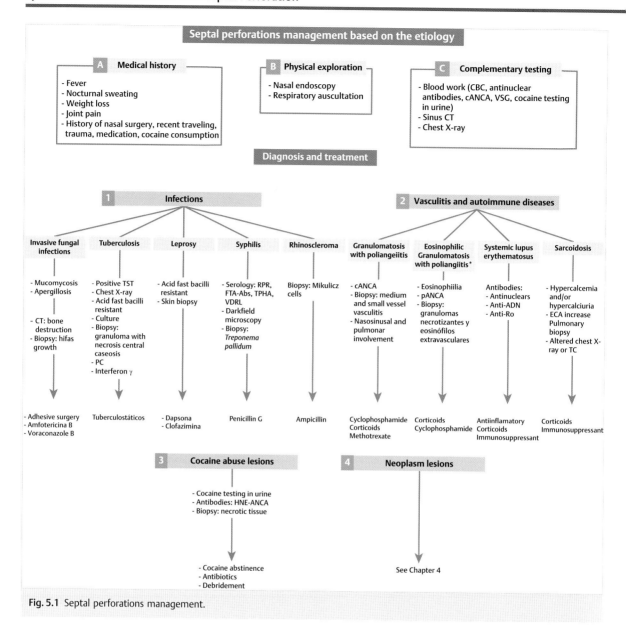

Fig. 5.1 Septal perforations management.

in all patients with advanced states of disease.[13,14] The nasal symptoms range from nosebleed, thick nasal discharge, ulcerations, septum perforations to total destruction of the nasal support causing the saddle-nose deformity, palate fistula, or even cavernous sinus thrombosis, a potentially fatal complication.[6,14]

The diagnosis of leprosy is based on clinical signs and symptoms. The observation of acid-fast bacteria in the skin-scraping examination confirms the diagnosis.

The recommended treatment of leprosy by the World Health Organization (WHO) includes dapsone, rifampin, and clofazimine.[15] The use of supervised multidrug therapy for fixed durations has been highly effective in treating all forms of the disease.[15]

5.1.3 Syphilis

Syphilis is an infectious disease caused by a spirochete called *Treponema pallidum* that has a tropism for several organs and tissues in the body causing complex clinical manifestations.[16]

In the United States approximately 6,000 cases are diagnosed each year of primary and secondary syphilis.[5] The incidence of syphilis reached an all-time low in 2000, with 2.1 cases per 100,000 persons in United States.[17] During the last 8 years a significant resurgence of this disease has been reported in several countries such as the United States, Canada, England, France, Spain, Ireland, Eastern Europe, Russia, and China.[17] It is estimated that

55,000 new infections occurred in 2014 in the United States.[17]

Primary syphilis has little nasal manifestations, although few cases of nasal vestibule chancre have been reported.[5] Secondary syphilis can manifest as acute rhinitis with abundant nasal discharge with important irritation of the nasal mucosa.[18] If the disease progresses to tertiary syphilis, there is an important nasal involvement characterized by gummata of the nose, septal perforations, and destruction of the nasal support with saddle-nose and important deformity.[18] Involvement of nasopharynx is very uncommon.

The diagnosis of syphilis is based on the clinical signs and symptoms, physical examination, lesion-based test (dark-field microscopy, fluorescent antibody staining), and nontreponemal (rapid plasma reagin [RPR], venereal disease research laboratory [VDRL]) or treponemal (fluorescent treponemal antibody absorption [FTA-ABS], immunoglobulin G, Western blot) serologic tests.[19] Microorganism detection is useless for the diagnosis.

The mainstay of syphilis treatment is parenteral penicillin G. Doxycycline is an alternative in patients with penicillin allergy.[19]

5.1.4 Human Immunodeficiency Virus

Acute and chronic rhinosinusitis may occur in patients with human immunodeficiency virus (HIV) due to humoral and cellular immunodeficiency and decreased ciliary clearance.[5] These patients may present with symptoms of nasal obstruction caused for nasopharyngeal hypertrophy (in the infection early stages), facial pain, smell alterations, rhinorrhea, and a postnasal drip. An exacerbation of allergic rhinitis is very common in HIV-infected patients.[5,20] Opportunistic infections, including fungal, viral, or mycobacterial infections that rarely occur in the immunocompetent patient, may occur.[5] Nasal polyps and nasal tumors, including lymphomas and Kaposi's sarcomas, have been reported in patients with AIDS.[21]

NSP in patients with HIV and AIDS has been attributed to varicella zoster and non-Hodgkin's lymphoma.[20] NSP due to *Histoplasma capsulatum* has been reported as presenting symptoms in patients with AIDS.[22] Few cases have been reported of patients with NSP primarily caused by AIDS.[20] Positive HIV antibodies are detected with ELISA (enzyme-linked immunosorbent assay) and the diagnosis is confirmed by analyzing the viral proteins with Western blot.[5]

The rapid antiretroviral therapy (ART) initiation improves immune function, reduces the size of the viral reservoir, and limits the risk of onward viral transmission.[23] Recent studies show that immediate ART has a clinical benefit over deferral of treatment according to CD4 count threshold.[23] The WHO currently recommends the immediate start of the therapy, irrespective of CD4 count, for all individuals living with HIV.[23]

5.1.5 Fungal Infections

Fungal sinusitis appears in immunocompromised patients. *Aspergillus* spp. and *Mucor* spp. are the most commonly involved fungi.[6] Patients usually present bloody nasal discharge, facial pain and swelling, fever, and edema.[24] The disease progresses rapidly to facial cellulitis, gangrenous mucosal changes in the nose, and paranasal sinuses resulting in nasal septum ulceration and perforation, cranial nerve palsies, vision loss, and proptosis with an intracranial extension.[24]

Patients with suspected rhinocerebral disease should undergo an emergent CT scanning of the paranasal sinuses and an endoscopic nasal examination with biopsies of any suggestive lesions (pale or gray mucosa of the nasal cavity or palate or black middle turbinate).[25] The diagnosis of mucormycosis is established by obtaining a biopsy specimen of the involved tissue (samples should be immediately evaluated for signs of infection).[25]

Treatment requires antifungal agents such as amphotericin B or posaconazole (second line) and an early aggressive surgical debridement.[6,25] Maintaining a high index of suspicion in at-risk patient populations, followed by prompt evaluation and management, is crucial in the reduction of mortality rate.[25]

5.2 Multisystemic Disorders (Vasculitis and Autoimmune Diseases)

The frequency of NSP in patients with multisystemic disorders is also unknown due to the scarce number of publications. In the following section, the most frequent multisystemic diseases associated with NSP are described.

5.2.1 Granulomatosis with Polyangiitis

Granulomatosis with polyangiitis (GPA) is a systemic, idiopathic disease described as a necrotizing, granulomatous inflammation involving the upper and lower respiratory tracts in combination with glomerulonephritis and systemic vasculitis.[5,6] GPA predominantly affects the walls of small to medium arteries and veins.[26] A limited form in the upper respiratory tract presenting a midline destructive lesion of the nose and sinuses has been described.[5] The peak incidence is in the fourth through sixth decades of life.[26] The estimated prevalence in the United States is between 13 and 30 cases per million persons per 5-year period. GPA is more common in northern Europe. Annual incidence rates per million of GPA were 12 in Norway, 10.3 in England, and 4.1 in Spain.[26] Nasal symptoms include obstruction, rhinorrhea, minor and recurrent epistaxis, crusting, and pain over the nasal dorsum.[6] Hyposmia may also occur by secretions in early stages. Nasal endoscopy reveals an erythematous, friable mucosa with crusting and granulation that predominates in the septum and inferior turbinate.[26] Patients with an aggressive GPA present nonvascular necrosis causing bone destruction initially affecting the nasal septum (NSP) and then spreading to the turbinate, antrum wall, ethmoid sinus, laminae papyracea, and cribriform plate with conservation of the hard palate.[27] Diamantopoulos II and Jones reported GPA as a cause of perforation in 6/54 patients.[27] In aggressive cases the destruction of the nasal support may lead to the characteristic saddle-nose deformity.[5,6,26]

The diagnosis is based on the combination of clinical symptoms, physical findings, radiologic examinations, laboratory testing (positive c-ANCA in 60–90%), and a biopsy of affected tissue.[5,6,26]

Treatment includes corticosteroids medication such as prednisone and cyclophosphamide or methotrexate.[5,6]

5.2.2 Eosinophilic Granulomatosis with Polyangiitis

Eosinophilic granulomatosis with polyangiitis (EGPA) is a rare small-sized vessel vasculitis with a prevalence of 1.3 cases per 100,000 inhabitants.[28] Systemic symptoms such as fever, fatigue, and weight loss are prominent.[29] Allergic rhinitis occurs in 75% of patients and usually is one of the first symptoms of EGPA.[29]

Diagnosis should be suspected in patients with asthma, with increased peripheral-blood eosinophil count and pulmonary infiltrates.[29] The American College of Rheumatology identified six major criteria for the diagnosis of the disease: asthma, peripheral neuropathy attributable to a systemic vasculitis, transient pulmonary infiltrates, paranasal sinus abnormality, peak blood peripheral eosinophilia of greater than 10%, and a biopsy specimen of a blood vessel with extravascular eosinophils.[5]

The syndrome is often associated with the presence of perinuclear antineutrophilic cytoplasmic antibodies that target mieloperoxidase.[28] Nasal polyps and recurrent sinusitis are present in approximately 50% of the patients.[5] Nasal pain with purulent or bloody nasal discharge, nasal crusting, or NSP is less common than in patients with GPA.[5]

Treatment usually includes high doses of corticosteroids and immunosuppressants such as cyclophosphamide.[29]

5.2.3 Sarcoidosis

Sarcoidosis is a chronic multisystemic disorder that usually affects young and middle-aged adults.[30] It is characterized by bilateral hilar lymphadenopathy, pulmonary infiltration, and ocular and skin lesions.[5] Studies show that sarcoidosis might be the result of an exaggerated granulomatous reaction after exposure to unidentified antigens in individuals who are genetically susceptible.[30]

A prevalence of 50 per 100,000 individuals has been reported.

The involvement of the epithelium of the upper respiratory tract is infrequent. The nasal symptoms are nonspecific: obstruction, epistaxis, nasal pain, epiphora, and anosmia.[6] The most consistent finding in the nose and sinuses is an erythematous, edematous, friable, hypertrophied mucosa predominantly in the septum and inferior turbinate. Submucosal nodules representative of intramucosal granulomas with a characteristic yellow color can be identified in mucosal biopsies.[5,31] Nasal polyposis, rhinophyma, and septal perforations have also been reported.[5] Aggressive noncaseating granulomas can cause hard or soft palate erosions as well as provoke a saddle-nose deformity.[32] Lawson et al classified sinonasal sarcoidosis in four subgroups: atrophic, hypertrophic, destructive, and nasal enlargement.[32]

The diagnosis of sarcoidosis of the nose and paranasal sinuses is based on the clinical findings with either polypoid changes or characteristic yellowish submucosal nodularity.[5] Tissue for diagnosis is usually obtained by transbronchial lung biopsy.[30] Other sites of biopsy are skin lesions, minor salivary glands, and lymph nodes.[5]

The primary treatment is systemic steroids,[32] although other treatments are chloroquine, immunosuppressors, and lung transplantation.[5,6,31,32]

5.2.4 Systemic Lupus Erythematosus

Systemic lupus erythematosus (SLE) is an autoimmune disease that can virtually affect any body system. SLE predominantly affects women (10:1). The incidence of SLE is 5.6 per 100,000 people, with an estimated prevalence of 130 per 100,000.[33]

SLE may have different symptoms such as extreme fatigue, painful or swollen joints (arthritis), unexplained fever, skin rashes, and kidney problems.[33] The skin of the nose and nasal vestibule can be involved in the skin rashes.[6] Mucosal lesions are seen in 9 to 18% of SLE cases with oral, nasal, and pharyngeal mucosae being most commonly affected.[33] Lisnevskaia et al reported six cases of patients with SLE and asymptomatic anterior NSP.[33]

Corticosteroid therapy or immunosuppressors are prescribed to control the symptoms.[5]

5.3 Conclusion

As described in this chapter, there exist a great variety of systemic and infectious diseases that can present with NSP, either at the beginning of the symptomatology or along the evolution of the clinical manifestations. Even though NSP is not a frequent presenting lesion, knowing the different etiologic entities will allow a proper medical management. An adequate medical history and a detailed physical examination are crucial for the correct orientation of the diagnosis in these patients. Complementary testing, including laboratory, imaging, and biopsies, also have a relevant role in this pathology involving very distinct etiologies.

References

[1] Nnadi CD, Anderson LF, Armstrong LR, et al. Mind the gap: TB trends in the USA and the UK, 2000–2011. Thorax. 2016; 71(4):356–363

[2] Casals M, Rodrigo T, Camprubí E, Orcau A, Caylà JA. [Tuberculosis and immigration in Spain: scoping review]. Rev Esp Salud Publica. 2014; 88(6):803–809

[3] Pareek M, Greenaway C, Noori T, Munoz J, Zenner D. The impact of migration on tuberculosis epidemiology and control in high-income countries: a review. BMC Med. 2016; 14(1):48

[4] Winston CA, Navin TR, Becerra JE, et al. Unexpected decline in tuberculosis cases coincident with economic recession—United States, 2009. BMC Public Health. 2011; 11:846

[5] Alobid I, Guilemany JM, Mullol J. Nasal manifestations of systemic illnesses. Curr Allergy Asthma Rep. 2004; 4(3):208–216

[6] Sardana K, Goel K. Nasal septal ulceration. Clin Dermatol. 2014; 32 (6):817–826

[7] Butt AA. Nasal tuberculosis in the 20th century. Am J Med Sci. 1997; 313(6):332–335

[8] Hup AK, Haitjema T, de Kuijper G. Primary nasal tuberculosis. Rhinology. 2001; 39(1):47–48

[9] Kaur R, Kachroo K, Sharma JK, Vatturi SM, Dang A. diagnostic accuracy of Xpert test in tuberculosis detection: a systematic review and meta-analysis. J Glob Infect Dis. 2016; 8(1):32–40

[10] Jian Y, Liu B, Guo L, Kong S, Su X, Lu C. [Pathogeny and treatment of 50 nasopharyngeal tuberculosis cases]. Lin Chung Er Bi Yan Hou Tou Jing Wai Ke Za Zhi. 2012; 26(24):1138–1140

[11] Nsagha DS, Bamgboye EA, Assob JCN, et al. Elimination of leprosy as a public health problem by 2000 AD: an epidemiological perspective. Pan Afr Med J. 2011; 9:4

[12] Chaptini C, Marshman G. Leprosy: a review on elimination, reducing the disease burden, and future research. Lepr Rev. 2015; 86(4):307–315

[13] McDougall AC, Rees RJ, Weddell AG, Kanan MW. The histopathology of lepromatous leprosy in the nose. J Pathol. 1975; 115 (4):215–226

[14] Barton RP. Clinical manifestation of leprous rhinitis. Ann Otol Rhinol Laryngol. 1976; 85(1 Pt 1):74–82

[15] Britton WJ, Lockwood DNJ. Leprosy. Lancet. 2004; 363(9416):1209–1219

[16] Ficarra G, Carlos R. Syphilis: the renaissance of an old disease with oral implications. Head Neck Pathol. 2009; 3(3):195–206

[17] Centers for Disease Control and Prevention (CDC). Primary and secondary syphilis—United States, 2000–2001. MMWR Morb Mortal Wkly Rep. 2002; 51(43):971–973

[18] Pletcher SD, Cheung SW. Syphilis and otolaryngology. Otolaryngol Clin North Am. 2003; 36(4):595–605, vi

[19] Clement ME, Okeke NL, Hicks CB. Treatment of syphilis: a systematic review. JAMA. 2014; 312(18):1905–1917

[20] Rejali SD, Simo R, Saeed AM, de Carpentier J. Acquired immune deficiency syndrome (AIDS) presenting as a nasal septal perforation. Rhinology. 1999; 37(2):93–95

[21] Fokkens WJ, Lund VJ, Mullol J, et al. European Position Paper on Rhinosinusitis and Nasal Polyps 2012. Rhinol Suppl 2012;(23):3 p preceding table of contents, 1–298

[22] Jaimes A, Muvdi S, Alvarado Z, Rodríguez G. Perforation of the nasal septum as the first sign of histoplasmosis associated with AIDS and review of published literature. Mycopathologia. 2013; 176(1–2): 145–150

[23] Fidler S, Fox J. Primary HIV infection: a medical and public health emergency requiring rapid specialist management. Clin Med (Lond). 2016; 16(2):180–183

[24] Middlebrooks EH, Frost CJ, De Jesus RO, Massini TC, Schmalfuss IM, Mancuso AA. Acute invasive fungal rhinosinusitis: a comprehensive update of CT findings and design of an effective diagnostic imaging model. AJNR Am J Neuroradiol. 2015; 36(8):1529–1535

[25] Payne SJ, Mitzner R, Kunchala S, Roland L, McGinn JD. Acute invasive fungal rhinosinusitis: a 15-year experience with 41 patients. Otolaryngol Head Neck Surg. 2016; 154(4):759–764

[26] Gubbels SP, Barkhuizen A, Hwang PH. Head and neck manifestations of Wegener's granulomatosis. Otolaryngol Clin North Am. 2003; 36 (4):685–705

[27] Diamantopoulos II, Jones NS. The investigation of nasal septal perforations and ulcers. J Laryngol Otol. 2001; 115(7):541–544

[28] Chaigne B, Dion J, Guillevin L, Mouthon L, Terrier B. Pathophysiology of eosinophilic granulomatosis with polyangiitis (Churg-Strauss). Rev Med Interne. 2016; 37(5):337–342

[29] Groh M, Pagnoux C, Baldini C, et al. Eosinophilic granulomatosis with polyangiitis (Churg-Strauss) (EGPA) Consensus Task Force recommendations for evaluation and management. Eur J Intern Med. 2015; 26(7):545–553

[30] Valeyre D, Prasse A, Nunes H, Uzunhan Y, Brillet P-Y, Müller-Quernheim J. Sarcoidosis. Lancet. 2014; 383(9923):1155–1167

[31] Judson MA. The clinical features of sarcoidosis: a comprehensive review. Clin Rev Allergy Immunol. 2015; 49(1):63–78

[32] Lawson W, Jiang N, Cheng J. Sinonasal sarcoidosis: A new system of classification acting as a guide to diagnosis and treatment. Am J Rhinol Allergy. 2014; 28(4):317–322

[33] Lisnevskaia L, Murphy G, Isenberg D. Systemic lupus erythematosus. Lancet. 2014; 384(9957):1878–1888

Chapter 6

Preoperative Clinical Evaluation of Patient

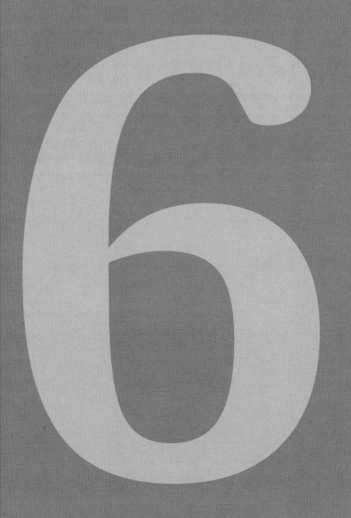

6 Preoperative Clinical Evaluation of Patient

Fabio Ferreli, Paolo Castelnuovo

Summary

A preoperative overview for nasal septal perforations requires both an anatomical local evaluation and specific diagnostic test. The assessment begins with carefully assessing patient's medical history. The physical examination starts with the inspection of the nasal pyramid for any alterations regarding the structural deficit. The nasal endoscopy allows the definition of the size and site of the perforation. The septum should be palpated with a sticker or with a cotton-tip in order to discern persistent cartilage between mucosal flaps and to determine whether cartilage extends close to the edges of the defect. CT scan with bone details can provide information about the structure of the residual septum and quantify the exact measurements of bone/cartilage defect. Lab tests should also be considered.

The causes of nasal septal perforations (NSPs) are numerous and can be either related to local or systemic conditions. Therefore, a preoperative overview requires both an anatomical local evaluation and specific diagnostic test.

It is essential, before proposing any surgical treatment, to clarify the etiopathogenesis of NSP.

The assessment begins with assessing the patient's medical history carefully. Patients may present the major symptoms of NSP, such as crusting, bleeding, whistling, nasal obstruction, and, sometimes, pain and rhinorrhea. It is necessary to investigate the onset of the NSP and any previous intranasal procedures eventually associated with septoplasty, and septal cauterization for anterior epistaxis. The possibility of septal damage can be linked to particular events, such as trauma, cocaine, nasal foreign-body injuries, and decubitus by nasogastric tube.

Some patients' habits can be considered, such as excessive use of nasal decongestants or topic steroid, and frequent digital trauma to remove intranasal crust. Finally, some risk factors related to occupational exposure, such as chemical irritants, and to specific diseases, for instance tuberculosis or syphilis, should be investigated.[1]

The physical examination starts with inspection of the nasal pyramid for any alterations regarding the structural deficit. Indeed, large NSP can result in loss of support of the nasal dorsum and consequent "saddle nose," sometimes associated with a deviation of the caudal edge of the septum. The nasal endoscopy with rigid fiber optics (30 degrees) is a key step of the physical examination. The use of topical decongestants and local anesthetics can make it easier and tolerable, especially in cases where the removal of crusts by an underlying mucosa, easily bleeding areas, or a biopsy is expected.

Upon physical examination of the nose, a full diagnosis cannot be made until all crusts have been removed and decongestion of the turbinates has taken place, making it possible to visualize the entire nasal septum. The nasal endoscopy allows appreciating the configuration of the NSP, the presence or absence of adherent crusts on the edges of the defect (▶ Fig. 6.1), any easily bleeding areas (▶ Fig. 6.2), and the state of the remaining mucosa, which may present some aspects regarding ischemic conditions (cocaine abuse) (▶ Fig. 6.3).

In addition, it is possible to measure the size of the NSP under endoscopic control that is critical when choosing the most suitable surgery (▶ Fig. 6.4).

The measurement of the defect can be performed in several ways.

The disposable paper ruler found in some surgical pen packs can be trimmed and introduced into the nose to obtain an accurate measurement. If this instrument is not available, the graduated end of the Cottle septum elevator can be carefully inserted and slid against the septum to determine the size of the NSP.

If the defect is not circular, but oval in shape (▶ Fig. 6.5), it is appropriate to obtain an exact measurement of the major diameters: anteroposterior and craniocaudal, vital in choosing the most appropriate surgical

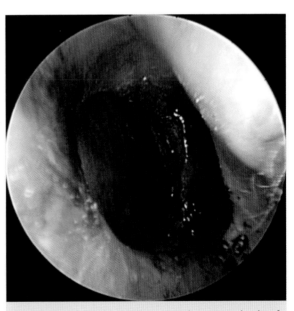

Fig. 6.1 The left nasal fossa. Crusting on the posterior border of septal perforation.

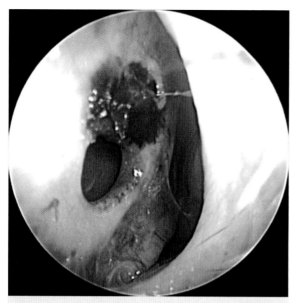

Fig. 6.2 The left nasal fossa. Small perforation with bleeding area.

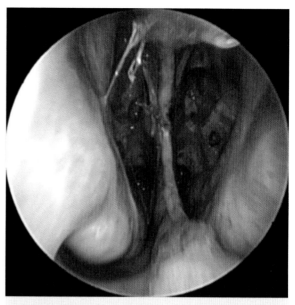

Fig. 6.3 The right nasal fossa. Large perforation in a cocaine user, with ischemic aspect of mucosa and infection.

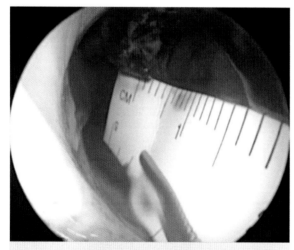

Fig. 6.4 The right nasal fossa. The septal perforation is measured with direct visualization during endoscopic examination.

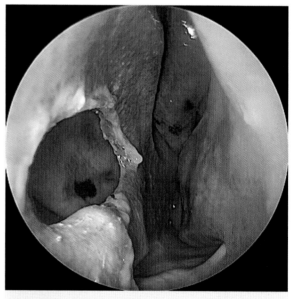

Fig. 6.5 The left nasal fossa. Septal perforation with oval shape.

technique. The vertical height of a perforation has been predicted to play a more important role in determining the surgical success than the horizontal length because the main tension between the floor of the nose and the dorsum was critical.[2] The final aspect that must be considered for surgery is the location: anterior, posterior, near the floor, or in the cranial part of the septum. Septal spurs must be identified during endoscopic examination. These should be removed during flap harvesting to get

one more large and flexible mucosal layer. Latter is an important aspect to achieve the NSP closure without tension (▶ Fig. 6.6). The septum should be palpated with a sticker or with a cotton tip to discern persistent cartilage between mucosal flaps and determine whether cartilage extends close to the edges of the NSP.[2] In perforations that have occurred after septoplasty, there is usually very little cartilage left, and this makes dissection of the flaps more difficult. In this phase it is also important to check

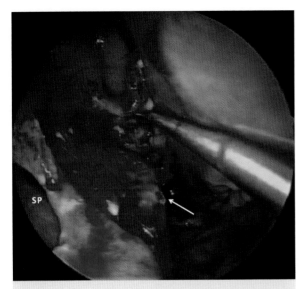

Fig. 6.6 The left nasal fossa. Septal spur (white arrow) posterior to the perforation. SP, septal perforation.

the quality of other intranasal anatomical structures, which represented potential donor sites of grafts or flaps, such as the inferior turbinate, the middle turbinate or the floor of the nasal fossa.

Often, the size of the bone or cartilage defect may be greater than the mucosal borders of NSP. Therefore, a radiologic investigation such as a computed tomographic (CT) scan with bone details can provide information about the structure of the residual septum and quantify the exact measurements of bone/cartilage defect. CT scans can also show any inflammation coexisting at the level of paranasal sinuses.

In patients without a likely local cause for the NSP or in patients with rheumatologic complaints, basic laboratory studies may be performed.

The rheumatoid factor (RF) level may be elevated in patients with rheumatoid arthritis, mixed connective tissue diseases, lupus, scleroderma, or other disorders. Elevated angiotensin-converting enzyme (ACE) levels can indicate the presence of sarcoidosis. Chest radiography can also be performed to assess mediastinal lymphadenopathies.

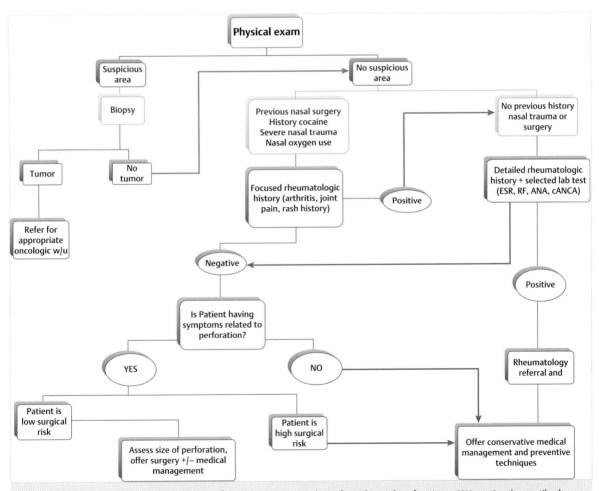

Fig. 6.7 Proposed algorithm modified by Batniji[5] for a systematic workup of nasal septal perforations. ANA, antinuclear antibody; c-ANCA, cytoplasmic antineutrophil cytoplasmic antibodies; ESR, erythrocyte sedimentation rate; RF, rheumatoid factor.

Churg-Strauss syndrome is characterized by increased levels of antineutrophil cytoplasmatic antibodies (p-ANCA) and eosinophilia. Wegener's granulomatosis is often associated with increased levels of antineutrophil cytoplasmatic antibodies (c-ANCA), erythrocyte sedimentation rate (ESR), and RF, but these are less specific indices.[3]

If any of the results are positive, consult a rheumatologist regarding further investigation.

For patients who use cocaine, it is absolutely mandatory to identify whether cocaine catabolizes in urine, or if possible, from hair. These patients must sustain or cease cocaine use at least 1 year prior to performing surgery. These patients should undergo periodic endoscopic controls to perform a toilet of the nasal cavity and remove the crusts from the edges of the perforation to prepare the surgical field. Moreover, instillation of drug emollients and antibiotic ointments are indicated.

In case of active and inflamed lesions of the septum around the mucosal edges of the perforation, a biopsy should be performed. The tissue can be sent for histopathological examination to exclude neoplastic lesions as well as for fungal and acid-fast bacilli cultures.

Biopsies of the superior edge of the NSP should be avoided because they contribute to increasing the cranio-caudal diameter as well as the difficulty in the surgical repair.[4]

Batniji in 2012 proposed an algorithm for the preoperative evaluation of the septal perforation,[5] which is shown in the flow chart in (▶ Fig. 6.7)

References

[1] Kridel RW. Considerations in the etiology, treatment, and repair of septal perforations. Facial Plast Surg Clin North Am. 2004; 12(4): 435–450, vi

[2] Kridel RW. Septal perforation repair. Otolaryngol Clin North Am. 1999; 32(4):695–724

[3] Diamantopoulos II, Jones NS. The investigation of nasal septal perforations and ulcers. J Laryngol Otol. 2001; 115(7):541–544

[4] Watson D, Barkdull G. Surgical management of the septal perforation. Otolaryngol Clin North Am. 2009; 42(3):483–493

[5] Batniji RK. Septal Perforation—Medical Aspects Treatment & Management. Medscape Reference Feb, 2012. emedicine.medscape.com

Chapter 7
Conservative Treatment

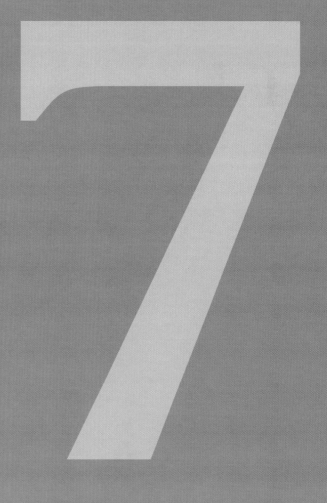

7 Conservative Treatment

Arturo Cordero Castillo, Mauricio López-Chacón, Cristobal Langdon, Isam Alobid

Summary

The most common causes of nasal septal perforation (NSP) are traumatic, postsurgical procedure, inflammatory diseases, and substance abuse. Between 1 and 39% of patients with NSP do not experience any symptoms and are diagnosed during a routine ENT (ear-nose-throat) examination. Conservative managements include nasal irrigation with isotonic saline, application of antibiotic and/ or vitamin ointment, or prosthesis such as a septal button. Surgical procedures are indicated when conservative treatment failed. This chapter focuses on the conservative management as a first-line treatment for those symptomatic cases, leaving surgical repairs for those who do not respond to conservative management.

7.1 Introduction

Nasal septal perforation (NSP) can occur by multiple etiologies, including previous trauma, iatrogenic, inflammatory diseases, substance abuse (e.g., cocaine), use of nasal spray, and others. The prevalence is believed to be approximately 1%; however, 39% of the patients remain asymptomatic until incidental diagnosis in a routine ENT examination. Although most patients with NSP remain asymptomatic, some suffer from bothersome symptoms such as epistaxis, crusting, sensation of nasal obstruction, pain, or discomfort—mostly associated with large perforations. The patients who are in the symptomatic group should initiate with a conservative treatment. If nasal moisture is preserved, the septal perforation is usually asymptomatic. Conservative managements include nasal irrigation with isotonic saline, application of antibiotic and/ or vitamin ointment, or prosthesis such as a septal button. If, despite this conservative management, patients still have bothersome symptoms that affect their quality of life, more aggressive treatments such as surgery can be proposed.

7.2 Pathogenesis

The nasal cavity receives its arterial supply from multiple branches that originated from both the internal and external carotid arteries. Of importance are the branches from the sphenopalatine, along with the superior labial artery, anterior ethmoidal artery (AEA), and greater palatine artery that nourish the Kiesselbach plexus, and therefore the anterior portion of the nasal septum, where most bleeding and perforation occur.[1,2,3,4,5,6]

A chemical or physical damage to the normal anatomy can lead to ischemic necrosis of the septal cartilage, resulting in perforation. Any healing result around the borders of the perforation over the three layers, cartilage, and the two sides of the mucoperichondrium is probably to be thin and atrophic. Therefore, if the edges of the perforation do not heal normally, it gets covered with an atrophic layer of mucosa, producing formation of crusts and a tendency toward bleeding because of the friction of abnormal airflow forces. The turbulent abnormal air forces friction, and the mechanical peeling to relieve a sensation of congestion may result in ongoing crusting, bleeding, and enlargement.[7]

When the septum is perforated, the inspired airflow going uniformly over the nasal turbinates adding heat and moisture to the air is disrupted. The inspired air loses its normal airflow pattern through the nasal cavity and begins to recirculate, producing excessive drying of the nasal mucosa that leads to its symptoms.

7.3 Symptoms

Despite being relatively uncommon, NSP has a varying presentation that may imitate pathologies such as septal deviation, allergic rhinitis, and, particularly, chronic rhinosinusitis, with which it may frequently coexist.[8] The patient perception of the symptoms may be influenced by the location and size of an NSP.[9] Diamantopoulos II and Jones[2] found that 92% of NSPs and ulcerations were located anteriorly and 8% were found posteriorly, and that those posterior lesions were frequently associated with trauma or systemic disease such as connective tissue disorders, neoplasia, and syphilis, whereas the anterior ones were associated with trauma and more symptomatic with bleeding and crusting.

The symptom most commonly reported by the patients was bleeding (58%), followed by crusting (43%), nasal obstruction (39%), pain (17%), and whistling (10%), with 15% being entirely asymptomatic, being whistling more often associated with a smaller NSP.[10] In larger NSP there is a great disturbance in laminar airflow and turbulence producing damage and drying of the respiratory epithelia; consequently, more rhinorrhea occurs as the nose attempts to improve the humidity. Turbulence may also create a nasal blockage sensation, which may lead to complications as the patient attempts to remove crusting by manual picking to improve congestion.[9]

Therefore, depending on the symptoms suffered by the patient will be the type of treatment recommended.

7.4 Conservative Treatment

The need for treatment depends on whether the patients have symptoms and indeed asymptomatic patients generally do not require any intervention. Underlying cause of septal perforation should be investigated before any intervention is taken. Consider the prevention of septal perforations in high-risk individuals (e.g., cocaine users).[11,12]

7.4.1 Saline Irrigation

Nasal douches are used in a variety of paranasal sinus diseases such as allergic rhinitis, chronic rhinosinusitis, follow-up treatment in paranasal sinus surgery, prevention in patients with recurrent nasal infection, and dry nose.[13,14]

According to the evidence, possible mechanism of action that improved mucosal function is due to a direct physical cleaning by irrigation of mucus, crusts, allergens, and debris, eliminating inflammation mediators, and improving the mucociliary clearance by enhancing the ciliary beating rate.[15,16,17,18]

Many different kinds of systems display into the market such as wash bottles (sinus rinse), Neti Pot, 60-cc catheter tip syringe, and baby bulb syringe. It can be found in many types of presentations, starting with the type of saline solution that goes from isotonic to hypertonic or the one that can be made at home. In general, most of them are isotonic solutions. Hypertonic saline irrigation not only acts on removing nasal secretions and crusting but also produces reversible cilia stasis, be it in vitro bactericidal and synergic with antibiotics. Osmotic pulls out edema from mucosa and may thin secretions.

Nasal irrigation can also have different pressures for every requirement (▶ Fig. 7.1). Those with low-flow volume go out nebulized allowing a soft cleaning and humidification of the nasal cavity, preferring as a maintenance therapy when there is no much secretion and crusts. The medium-flow volume is recommended when wanting a thorough cleaning or there are some crusts, leaving the high-flow volume for severe crusting and secretions. For irrigation of the whole nasal cavity, compressible douching systems that have a minimum output pressure of 120 mbar, a good connection of the outlet to the nostril, and irrigation stream that is directed upward (45 degrees) are recommended (▶ Fig. 7.2). Moreover, the material should be transparent, easy to clean, and disinfect, and should not contain harmful elements.[18]

7.4.2 Ointments

Nasal ointments exist with different components, the majority being formed by antibiotics and/or vitamin supplements. As it is known, while there is a septal perforation, the nasal mucosa tends to remain dry, and instead of producing more aqueous mucus to maintain a moist environment, it reduces its secretions. The secretion becomes sticky and mold of crusts are formed at the nasal septum when the air passes through the nasal cavity. When those crusts are released themselves, they may cause bleeding and new crust formation entering in a vicious cycle. Nasal ointments can protect the nasal mucosa from drying out, maintain nasal humidity, and reduce crusts formation, helping regeneration of the irritated and damaged mucosa, thus improving nasal congestion.

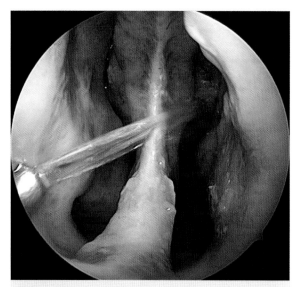

Fig. 7.1 Endoscopic endonasal view of nasal douches in an anterior nasal perforation.

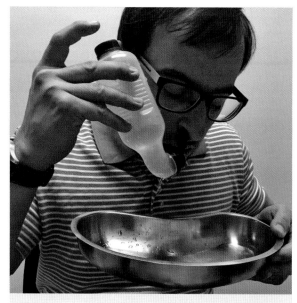

Fig. 7.2 Nasal irrigation with a compressible douching system.

The continuous production and release of crust may produce superinfection of the nasal mucosa, being useful in this cases an antibiotic ointment. Nasal cream instillation with antibiotic (e.g., Bactroban and Naseptin) can keep the edges of the perforation moist, minimizing crusting formation, nasal blockage, and treating and preventing infections.

7.4.3 Nasal Packs

Nasal packing should be used in the cases where hemostatic a reabsorbable agent cannot control epistaxis. They are most commonly made of polyvinyl acetate (e.g., Merocel) and should be used. If necessary, use those with smooth surface to minimize mucosal damage, potential worsening of wound healing, and negative impact on patient comfort.[19]

7.4.4 Hemostatic and/or Reabsorbable Agents

The ideal nasal dressing is one that is hemostatic, absorbable, and favors healing. Although most of the currently available materials may have one of these characteristics, none presents all.[20]

Currently available dressings include the following:
1. Denatured porcine collagen: Lyostypt, Diacoll
2. Hyaluronic acid: Merocel
3. Oxidized regenerated cellulose: Surgicel
4. Carboxy-Methyl-Cellulosa: Stammberger foam, Rapid Rhino
5. Hemostatics gels with thrombin: Floseal, Crosseal
6. Polysaccharides as Chitosan gel, promoted by Wormald-Medtronic

7.5 Symptom-Based Treatment

Symptoms-based treatments are listed in ▶ Table 7.1.

7.5.1 Epistaxis

Epistaxis is considered the most common symptom (58%) in the majority of series (58%).[21] As in any other epistaxis, the first step is to rule out an underlying cause such as hypertension, vasculitic associated diseases, and medications that influence in the coagulation (e.g., acetylsalicylic acid), and treat it before any intervention is taken. If required, it may use different types of packing or hemostatics. Whenever possible, the use of resorbable hemostatic agents (e.g., Merocel, Surgicel, Rapid Rhino) is preferred; however, if the bleeding is not controlled, nasal packing is recommended for 48 to 72 hours. After removing the packing, it is necessary to make nasal irrigation. Force is decided depending on the symptoms and crusting, and nasal ointments after irrigations.

7.5.2 Crusting and Nasal Congestion

Series have reported crusting in 43% and nasal congestion in 35%, making them important symptoms in nasal perforations.[21] Treatment is focused depending on the amount of crusting and congestion that the patient refers, being the nasal irrigation and nasal ointment the mainstays treatments. In general, the use of high-flow volume irrigation for severe crusting and congestion and medium-flow volume for the rest of the patients is recommended, leaving low-flow volumes for maintenance. Nasal ointments are used after nasal irrigation. If suspect of infection, an antibiotic ointment is preferred. If that is not the case, a nonantibiotic ointment should be used as a maintenance or long-lasting therapy.

7.5.3 Conclusion

The need for treatment depends on whether the patient is experiencing symptoms; however, as most cases of the NSP remain asymptomatic, no treatment is required. In symptomatic patients the first step is to manage the underlying cause and encourage a possible natural healing before any intervention is taken. In those symptomatic cases conservative treatment should be initiated with nasal douches and ointments helping to ameliorate the symptoms and decrease its complications by keeping the edges of the perforation moist. Other conservative

Table 7.1 Symptom-based treatment

	Symptoms	Treatment
Epistaxis	Mild/moderated	• Resorbable hemostatic agents • Nasal irrigation with low/moderate flow volumes • Vitamin nasal ointment
	Severe	• Nasal packing
Crusting	Mild	• Nasal irrigation with low flow volumes • Vitamin nasal ointments after each irrigation
	Moderated	• Nasal irrigation with medium flow volume • Vitamin nasal ointments after each irrigation
	Severe	• Nasal irrigation with high-flow volume • Vitamin nasal ointments after each irrigation
		• If suspect of infection, it is preferred an antibiotic ointment
Nasal obstruction		• Nasal irrigation with hypertonic saline solution • Vitamin nasal ointments after each irrigation

interventions include nasal packing, haemostatic, and reabsorbable agents.

In the cases that remain symptomatic despite conservative management, surgical treatment may be an option.

References

[1] Oberg D, Akerlund A, Johansson L, Bende M. Prevalence of nasal septal perforations: the Skovde population-based study. Rhinology. 2003; 41(2):72–75

[2] Diamantopoulos II, Jones NS. The investigation of nasal septal perforations and ulcers. J Laryngol Otol. 2001; 115(7):541–544

[3] Wong S, Raghavan U. Outcome of surgical closure of nasal septal perforation. J Laryngol Otol. 2010; 124(8):868–874

[4] Blind A, Hulterström A, Berggren D. Treatment of nasal septal perforations with a custom-made prosthesis. Eur Arch Otorhinolaryngol. 2009; 266(1):65–69

[5] Moon IJ, Kim SW, Han DH, et al. Predictive factors for the outcome of nasal septal perforation repair. Auris Nasus Larynx. 2011; 38(1):52–57

[6] Mercurio GA, Jr. Anatomic considerations of nasal blood supply. Ear Nose Throat J. 1981; 60(10):443–446

[7] Lanier B, Kai G, Marple B, Wall GM. Pathophysiology and progression of nasal septal perforation. Ann Allergy Asthma Immunol. 2007; 99(6):473–479, quiz 480–481, 521

[8] Bhattacharyya N. Clinical symptomatology and paranasal sinus involvement with nasal septal perforation. Laryngoscope. 2007; 117(4):691–694

[9] Brain DJ. Septo-rhinoplasty: the closure of septal perforations. J Laryngol Otol. 1980; 94(5):495–505

[10] Kuriloff DB. Nasal septal perforations and nasal obstruction. Otolaryngol Clin North Am. 1989; 22(2):333–350

[11] Mullace M, Gorini E, Sbrocca M, Artesi L, Mevio N. Management of nasal septal perforation using silicone nasal septal button. Acta Otorhinolaryngol Ital. 2006; 26(4):216–218

[12] Pedroza F, Patrocinio LG, Arevalo O. A review of 25-year experience of nasal septal perforation repair. Arch Facial Plast Surg. 2007; 9(1):12–18

[13] Harvey R, Hannan SA, Badia L, Scadding G. Nasal saline irrigations for the symptoms of chronic rhinosinusitis. Cochrane Database Syst Rev. 2007; 18(3):CD006394

[14] Hildenbrand T, Weber R, Heubach C, Mösges R. [Nasal douching in acute rhinosinusitis]. Laryngorhinootologie. 2011; 90(6):346–351

[15] Georgitis JW. Nasal hyperthermia and simple irrigation for perennial rhinitis. Changes in inflammatory mediators. Chest. 1994; 106(5):1487–1492

[16] Boek WM, Keleş N, Graamans K, Huizing EH. Physiologic and hypertonic saline solutions impair ciliary activity in vitro. Laryngoscope. 1999; 109(3):396–399

[17] Talbot AR, Herr TM, Parsons DS. Mucociliary clearance and buffered hypertonic saline solution. Laryngoscope. 1997; 107(4):500–503

[18] Campos J, Heppt W, Weber R. Nasal douches for diseases of the nose and the paranasal sinuses—a comparative in vitro investigation. Eur Arch Otorhinolaryngol. 2013; 270(11):2891–2899

[19] Weber RK. [Nasal packing and stenting]. Laryngorhinootologie. 2009; 88 Suppl 1:S139–S155

[20] Valentine R, Wormald PJ. Nasal dressings after endoscopic sinus surgery: what and why? Curr Opin Otolaryngol Head Neck Surg. 2010; 18(1):44–48

[21] Kridel RW. Considerations in the etiology, treatment, and repair of septal perforations. Facial Plast Surg Clin North Am. 2004; 12(4):435–450, vi

Chapter 8

Nasal Perforation and Septal Prosthesis

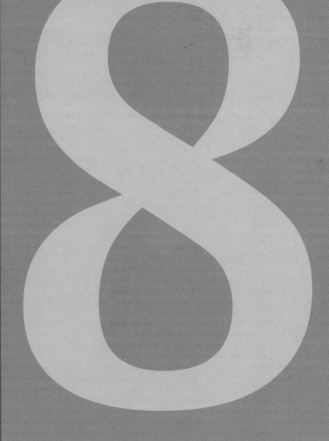

8 Nasal Perforation and Septal Prosthesis

Meritxell Valls, Alfonso Santamaría, Isam Alobid

Summary

Surgical repair of a nasal septal perforation is a complex situation for which many different techniques have been described in this book. This suggests that there is no single ideal procedure. Nonsurgical closure of nasal perforation can be achieved with a simple technique inserting a preformed or a custom-made prosthesis. Not all patients tolerate the presence of a nasal foreign body; however, many find it more acceptable than their symptoms before insertion of the obturator.

8.1 Anatomy

The nasal septum divides the nose into two similar halves. The majority of the anterior septum is made up by the quadrangular cartilage. The posterior aspect of the septum is predominantly bony and includes the perpendicular plate of the ethmoid bone superiorly and the vomer inferiorly. The nasal septum might present deviation or other deformities that should be taken into account given that it could complicate the adaptation of a nasal prosthesis in a septal perforation.

8.2 Indications

- Symptomatic small and large nasal septal perforations.
- Patients with contraindication for surgical approach to repair the perforation.
- Patients who refuse further surgical approaches.
- The perforation must have a complete circumferential ridge of nasal septal tissue around the perforation to support the prosthesis.

8.3 Materials

Tolerance of nasal septal prosthesis may be influenced by the type of material. The initial nylon and Luxene prosthetics have been replaced by more biocompatible silicone elastomer and acrylic ones.[1] Silicone currently constitutes most prefabricated prosthetics—as seen in 20 (87%) of 23 of this systematic review's case series—whereas acrylic prosthetic outcomes were presented in only one case study, involving a custom, two-piece, magnetized heat-processed acrylic resin.[2] It has been theorized that acrylic may be the preferred material as

silicone's porous structure may sorb comparably more mucus, leading to greater crusting, surrounding tissue irritation, and patient discomfort. It has been proposed that silicone may deteriorate more over time than acrylic due to its lesser inherent physical strength.[3]

However, these speculations are unable to be assessed at the present time due to the paucity of data on acrylic prosthetics. Prosthetic construction may influence patient comfort and symptom improvement. There are prefabricated prosthetics models in one and two pieces. The two-piece models may facilitate insertion by the surgeon and regular cleaning by the patient. Though this cleaning offers the advantage of less crust accumulation on the prosthetic, there are reports of patients discontinuing their use due to difficult reinsertion after cleaning.[4]

8.3.1 Prefabricated versus Custom Made

In a recent review no studies were found directly comparing prefabricated prosthetics with custom-made ones.[1] In general, custom-made prosthetics are the preferred choice for symptomatic perforations of large size (≥ 2 cm), posterior or basal location, or irregular edges.[4,5,6] The mentioned characteristics increase the likelihood of an imprecise fit, which may contribute to greater crusting, nasal obstruction, foreign-body sensation, mucosal necrosis, prosthetic migration, and prosthetic loss.[1] Septal defect can be outlined using aluminum foil, blotting paper, or measured by computed tomographic (CT) scan to design the custom-made prosthetic. With these techniques, personalized prosthetics can accommodate variations in septal thickness better than prefabricated prosthetics and are comparatively more fixed in place by their contour. These features theoretically minimize crust buildup, which can be further reduced by using removable custom prosthetics, such as those described by Blind et al or magnet-attached two-piece prosthetics.[7] The main limitation of custom prosthetics is that they require a prosthetist to construct them, leading to longer operative times and greater costs than prefabricated prosthetics.

8.4 Surgical Steps

Positioning of nasal prosthetics can be performed under local or general anesthesia, but generally local anesthesia is preferred. In this chapter we illustrate one of the possible methods to place a conventional one-piece Silastic button.

1. Topical nasal decongestion and anesthesia. Infiltration of the anterior septum, floor of the nose, and surroundings of the perforation with a solution of lidocaine and epinephrine (1:100.000) to achieve correct homeostasis and anesthesia.

2. Ensure to de-crust the edges of the perforation meticulously to expose it completely.

3. The perforation can be measured by placing a template (e.g., a piece of card or white paper) on the one side and marking the perforation from the other side. The template should be correctly placed against the nasal septum. A cotton swab dipped in methylene blue can be used to mark the shape and size of the perforation, so that a bespoke button can be shaped to the individual septal perforation[8] (► Fig. 8.1).

4. Carefully remove the card from the nasal cavity and cut the dyed part to assess the real size of the septal perforation. Then place it over the septal button as a template. Disks may be trimmed but must remain larger than the perforation, so cut the septal button (silicone Silastic button) around the marked perforation area leaving an appropriate margin (3–5 mm beyond the edge of the nasal perforation) (► Fig. 8.2).

5. To make easier the insertion of the septal button, use a purse-string suture technique with 2–0 silk suture to collapse one disk of the Silastic obturator with approximately 8-mm spaces between each puncture site (► Fig. 8.3a), as described by Kelly and Lee.[9]

6. Tie the suture and the Silastic disc will fold over itself. The silk suture is then looped around the folded flange and a second knot is tied, which further collapses the disk (► Fig. 8.3b).

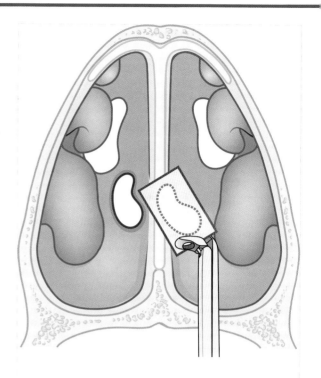

Fig. 8.1 This drawing exemplifies one possible method for determining the exact shape and size of the septal perforation. A piece of cardboard is used as a template and introduced into the left nasal cavity attached to the septum. From the right nasal cavity, the edges of the perforation are marked with a cotton swab dipped in methylene blue obtaining a custom-made template that will be used to shape the button to the individual septal perforation.

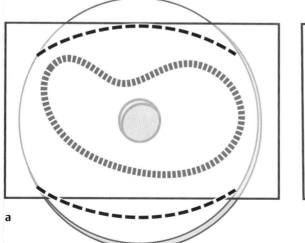

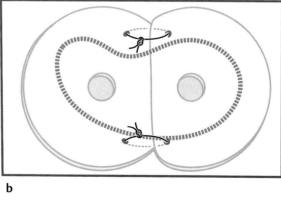

a

b

Fig. 8.2 Modifications of the septal button/s. Template of the septal perforation dyed in methylene blue. **(a)** The disks may be trimmed but must remain larger than the perforation, so cut the septal button (red marks) around the marked perforation area leaving an appropriate margin (3–5 mm beyond the edge of the nasal perforation). **(b)** Drawing of a double septal button. If the perforation is too large to be covered up for one single button, it is possible to cut and suture two of them to cover the perforation fully (Illing, 2012).

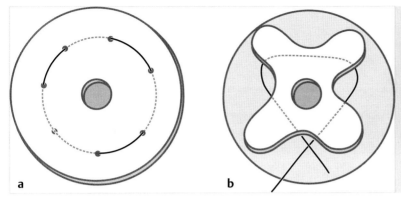

Fig. 8.3 (a) Purse-string suture technique with 2–0 silk suture with approximately 8-mm spaces between each puncture site. The entrance and exit of the suture should be placed in the medial aspect of the Silastic flange. **(b)** Tie the suture and automatically the disk will fold up. Then loop the suture around the folded flange to narrow even more this half of the septal button.

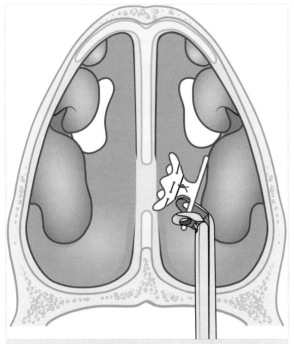

Fig. 8.4 Introduction of the septal button into the nasal cavity. The unfolded disk of the Silastic button is grasped with a Tilley or a Blakesley forceps and introduced into one nasal cavity. The collapsed disk is advanced through the septal perforation under endoscopic vision.

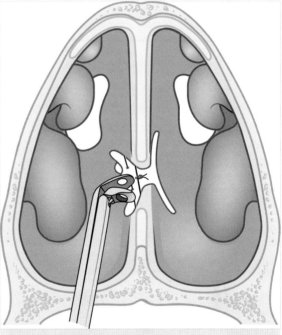

Fig. 8.5 Introduction of the septal button into the perforation. From the contralateral nasal cavity, grasp the folded flange of the septal button and pull to fit it into the septal perforation avoiding damaging the septal mucosa.

7. Lubricate the button. The other disk of the Silastic button is then grasped with forceps and introduced into one nasal cavity. The collapsed disk is advanced through the septal perforation under direct headlight illumination or endoscopic ally (▶ Fig. 8.4).
8. Grasp the folded flange of the septal button with a clamp through the contralateral side and pull to fit it into the septal perforation (▶ Fig. 8.5). Once in place, the suture is cut allowing the Silastic disk to fold out and return to its original shape (▶ Fig. 8.6, ▶ Fig. 8.7a, b).
9. Ensure the flanges fit against the upper lateral cartilage–septum junction, and avoid pressure against the septal floor.

Thomas et al[10] described a different insertion technique: performing a circular slit starting from the outer edge of one of the flanges of the one-piece septal button. The slit

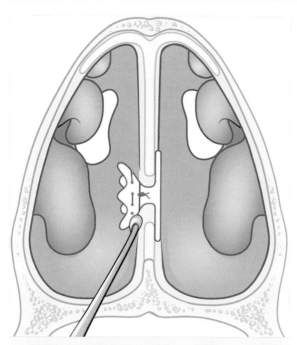

Fig. 8.6 Cut the suture allowing the Silastic disk to fold out and return to its original shape.

Blind et al[4] described this custom-made nasal septal silicone prosthesis. The shape of the prosthesis is made from an alginate mold, an adequate material to give a very detailed template and delicate with the sensitive nasal mucosa (▶ Fig. 8.8). The prosthesis is grasped from the handle and introduced from one side and fit into the nasal septal perforation with little discomfort because of the soft and elastic material. The central part of the button is thinned down to maximize breathing through the nose. When in place, the handle will be hidden under the alar dome (▶ Fig. 8.9a, b). This system allows the patient and the physician to remove and reinsert the prosthesis easily. The main disadvantage is the technical difficulty of molding the prosthesis, as it usually requires cooperation of a dental prosthetist and specialized materials.

8.5 Postoperative Care

Proper nasal hygiene plays a vital role in success and requires patient cooperation. Nasal irrigation is encouraged three times a day followed by topic vitamin A ointment that helps hydrate and regenerate nasal mucosa after septal button insertion.

8.6 Discussion

Although surgical closure should always be considered first as the best therapy option, septal perforation surgery has some disadvantages—the main being difficulty in effectively closing the septal perforation, which is directly related to the size of the defect. Another problem is the

goes in toward the hub covering 300 degrees of the circle of the flange. Then split end of the flange is pulled through the perforation into the other nasal cavity. By rotating the button, all of the flange will be in the other nostril, and thus the button will be positioned accurately.

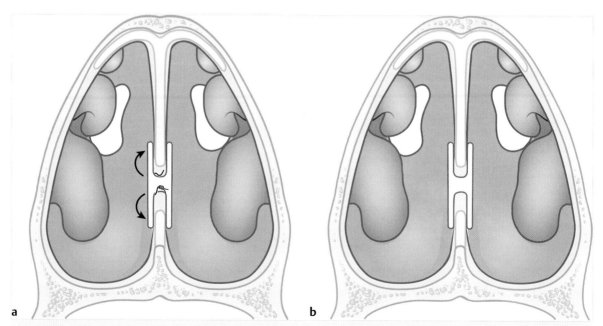

a

b

Fig. 8.7 (a) Septal button unfolding after cutting the sutures. **(b)** Septal button correctly placed covering the septal perforation completely.

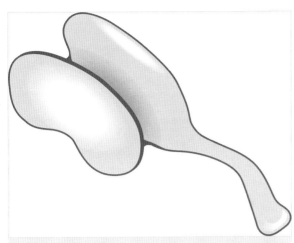

Fig. 8.8 Custom-made nasal septal silicone prosthesis described by Blind et al.[4] This piece is manufactured to be inserted from the left nasal cavity. The central part is thinned to avoid interfering with nasal breathing.

acrylic and plastic in the past but are now primarily made of soft silicone. Prefabricated buttons are typically two-piece units with a flexible hub and pliable disks allowing them to adapt to the curvatures of the septum.[14] Also available are two-piece units, which tend to have greater ease of insertion. Buttons may be placed as temporary or long-term treatment and do not preclude future surgical closure. Nasal prosthesis for septal perforation is also an option for the patients in whom surgery may be contra-indicated because of age, comorbidities, or underlying pathology.

Custom-designed and prefabricated prosthetics have been described, with prefabricated models having the advantage of decreased operative time but the potential disadvantage of imprecise fit.[1] Prosthetics can be placed in the outpatient facility with or without local anesthesia or in the operating room under general anesthesia, depending on surgeon preference, patient-specific fac-tors, and type of prosthetic used. Surgical closure is diffi-cult in larger perforations and has the risk of failure. In these cases septal prosthesis is an effective alternative. Prosthetic closure can be achieved using prefabricated buttons or personalized obturators.[6]

However, they also have potential adverse effects: increase in epistaxis, pain and discomfort, erosion of the edges of the perforation, and they may serve as a site for crust deposition[5] (▶ Fig. 8.10). Patient intolerance occurs usually due to local irritation, nasal obstruction, or

fact that an unsuccessful operation can result in a larger perforation.[11] The use of composite grafts and prostheses has been reported to achieve good results.[12,13]

Among nonsurgical options to treat nasal septal perfo-ration, there are prosthetics, including buttons and other obturators, which close the defect mechanically without requiring tissue disruption. Buttons have been made from

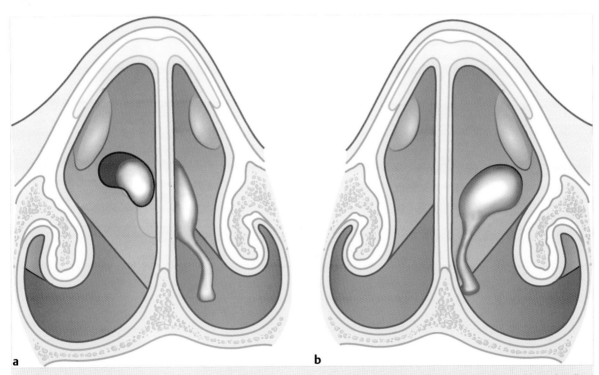

a b

Fig. 8.9 (a) Insertion of the nasal silicone prosthesis from the left nasal cavity without clamps; the prosthesis is grasped by its handle. (b) View from the left nasal cavity once the prosthesis is well placed. In this drawing the prosthesis is shown in purple to highlight from the background but normally is made in pink or red color to match the nasal mucosa.

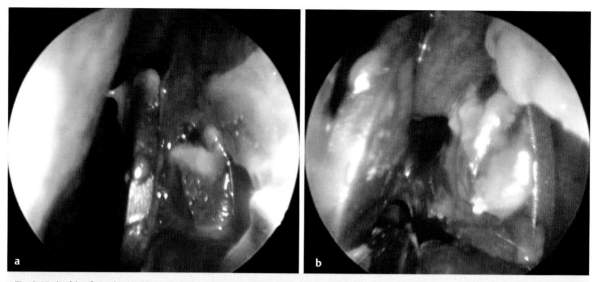

Fig. 8.10 (a, b) Infected septal button with secretions and crusts seen from the right nasal cavity.

accumulation of thick secretions. Patients who request removal usually do so within 6 months.[15] Difficult reinsertion of the prostheses may also lead to chronic irritation at the perforation borders that can enlarge the perforation over time and cause prosthetic dislodgement.[7] The risk for this is increased in an ill-fitting prosthetic, which is the primary limitation of prefabricated models.

Luff et al[16] studied 14 patients who underwent insertion of a septal button between 1990 and 2000 with a specific questionnaire and only 45% of patients maintained their button in a cumulative follow-up period of 10 years. On the other side, Eliachar and Mastros[14] and Mullace et al[17] report that 70% of patients remain with their nasal obturator in situ. Federspil and Schneider[18] presented a series of 57 patients with septal button followed during 7 years and 75% of the patients kept using the button after all those years with a high level of satisfaction. Artal et al[19] studied 22 patients with septal perforation treated with nasal buttons and reported 100% improvement in nasal obstruction and whistling, but only 59% of the patients ameliorated nasal dryness and crusting.

The systematic review recently conducted by Taylor and Sherris[1] reported that prosthetics were well tolerated and that the nasal symptoms improved in patients with perforations secondary to cocaine abuse,[17] systemic lupus erythematosus, and bevacizumab treatment. Other reported etiologies of nasal septal perforation such as Wegener's granulomatosis, sarcoidosis, malignant granuloma, tuberculosis, and Rendu-Osler-Weber disease have also been treated with a nasoseptal prosthetic, but the outcomes of these individual cases were not specified.

Several recent studies have examined outcomes when using CT with reformatted images to obtain a three-dimensional (3D) image of the defect to custom-fit septal

buttons. These techniques are particularly useful for large (>3 cm) perforations in which adjacent soft tissue to secure the button in place is limited. A precise fit is necessary to avoid movement of the button, which can enlarge the perforation and allow the button to be dislodged.[5] Additionally, CT-fabricated buttons may improve symptoms to a greater degree than traditional obturators.[6] Other recently described techniques for generating a custom-fit septal button prosthetics include a handled silicone-colored septal button prosthesis fashioned using an alginate mold and plaster cast[4] and a magnet-based two-piece button prosthesis (▶ Fig. 8.11).[7] Teschner et al[7] described the replacement procedure as not unpleasant for the patient because it allows to clean the button at short and regular time intervals and the patient has to do so on his or her own. On the other hand, Illing et al[20] described the "double septal button" method for dealing with large septal perforations, where a standard septal button would be of suboptimal fit and at high risk of dislodgement and ongoing symptoms. Patients should be warned that the prosthetic may loosen or dislodge due to sneezing. In this sense, custom prosthetics can adapt variations in septal thickness better than prefabricated

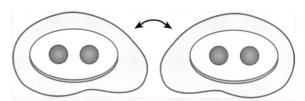

Fig. 8.11 Two-piece magnet-based septal button. The drawing shows the two corresponding halves of the nasal septal button. Because of the magnetic system, the device is easy to reinsert in case of dislodgement.

prosthetics and are comparatively more fixed in place by their contour, but the counterpart is that they require a prostheticist to construct them, leading to longer operative times and greater costs than prefabricated prosthetics.[1]

The systematic review of six low-risk-of-bias studies mentioned before[1] showed that literature provides considerable level 4 evidence for the efficacy and safety of prosthetics for nasal septal perforation treatment. This meta-analysis reports success rate of 65%. In the 706 cases that were reported in the literature, only 1 fungal infection and 9 unspecified infections were described. Price et al observed 74% success rates in 30 perforations greater than 3 cm, using custom one-piece silicone prosthetics designed from sagittal CT,[5] which compares favorably to reported surgical success rates of 78% for perforations greater than 2 cm.[21] On the contrary, Døsen and Haye reported 67% removal of the septal button in a study with long observation period (mean 13 years). They describe that large perforations and those that are due to septal resection (Killian) are associated with a poor prognosis.[22]

8.7 Points of Difficulty and Technical Solutions

Points of difficulty and technical solutions are shown in ▶ Table 8.1.

8.8 Case Example

A 60-year-old man with history of septal surgery 5 years ago presented with an anterior symptomatic nasal septal perforation. The main complaint was frequent episodes of epistaxis, crusts, and nasal obstruction. Conservative

Table 8.1 Points of difficulty and technical solutions

Points of difficulty	Technical solutions
Adaptation of the prosthesis to the shape and size of nasal septal perforation	Measure the septal defect ideally with a template as described in surgical steps. Cut the prefabricated prosthesis smoothly without sharp edges, leaving 3–5 mm beyond the size of the perforation.
Damaging the inferior turbinate	When inserting the prosthesis, be careful to stay near the septum and control endoscopically both sides, avoiding injuries to the inferior turbinate.
Insertion of the nasal prosthesis	In the case of the nasal silicone button, try the purse-string technique described in text. In other custom-made prosthesis, make sure it fits perfectly the nasal septal perforation and make it in a soft pliable material, allowing an easy and atraumatic insertion.

treatment with nasal douche and emollients did not improve his symptoms. On nasal endoscopy, a perforation of 2 cm diameter was found with complete circumferential ridge of nasal septal tissue around the perforation. He refused surgery so we offered the insertion of a Silastic button as a nonsurgical option.

Before insertion of the nasal septal button, the nasal cavity was decongested under local anesthesia with a solution of lidocaine and epinephrine (1:100.000). The prosthesis was molded to the size and shape of patient's perforation and inserted under endoscopic vision as indicated in Surgical Steps section.

8.9 Tips and Tricks

- Easy procedure under local or general anesthesia.
- Folding one of the flanges of the septal button with securing sutures reduces the surface area of the button and also makes the inserting edge narrower, facilitating easy insertion.
- Outcomes improve in custom-made prosthesis and are related with adequate postoperative care and cleaning.

References

References in bold are recommended readings.

[1] **Taylor RJ, Sherris DA. Prosthetics for nasal perforations: a systematic review and meta-analysis. Otolaryngol Head Neck Surg. 2015; 152(5):803–810**

[2] Sashi Purna CR, Annapurna PD, Ahmed SB, Vurla S, Nalla S, Abhishek SM. Two-piece nasal septum prosthesis for a large nasal septum perforation: a clinical report. J Prosthodont. 2013; 22(2):143–147

[3] Zaki HS, Myers EN. Prosthetic management of large nasal septal defects. J Prosthet Dent. 1997; 77(3):335–338

[4] **Blind A, Hulterström A, Berggren D. Treatment of nasal septal perforations with a custom-made prosthesis. Eur Arch Otorhinolaryngol. 2009; 266(1):65–69**

[5] Price DL, Sherris DA, Kern EB. Computed tomography for constructing custom nasal septal buttons. Arch Otolaryngol Head Neck Surg. 2003; 129(11):1236–1239

[6] Barraclough JP, Ellis D, Proops DW. A new method of construction of obturators for nasal septal perforations and evidence of outcomes. Clin Otolaryngol. 2007; 32(1):51–54

[7] Teschner M, Willenborg K, Lenarz T. Preliminary results of the new individual made magnet-based nasal septal button. Eur Arch Otorhinolaryngol. 2012; 269(3):861–865

[8] Ashraf N, Thevasagayam MS. Sizing a nasal septal button using a methylene blue-marked template. Clin Otolaryngol. 2015; 40(4):402

[9] Kelly G, Lee P. A new technique for the insertion of a Silastic button for septal perforations. Laryngoscope. 2001; 111(3):539–540

[10] Thomas L, Kalra G, Al-waa A, Karkanevatos A. Septal button insertion—the screw technique. Laryngoscope. 2010; 120(2):280–281

[11] Brain D. The nasal septum. In: Kerr AG, ed. Scott-Brown's Otolaryngology. London, UK: Butterworth; 1987:154–157

[12] Woolford TJ, Jones NS. Repair of nasal septal perforations using local mucosal flaps and a composite cartilage graft. J Laryngol Otol. 2001; 115(1):22–25

[13] Hussain A, Murthy P. Modified tragal cartilage–temporoparietal and deep temporal fascia sandwich graft technique for repair of nasal septal perforations. J Laryngol Otol. 1997; 111(5):435–437

[14] Eliachar I, Mastros NP. Improved nasal septal prosthetic button. Otolaryngol Head Neck Surg. 1995; 112(2):347–349

[15] Pallanch JF, Facer GW, Kern EB, Westwood WB. Prosthetic closure of nasal septal perforations. Otolaryngol Head Neck Surg. 1982; 90(4): 448–452

[16] Luff DA, Kam A, Bruce IA, Willatt DJ. Nasal septum buttons: symptom scores and satisfaction. J Laryngol Otol. 2002; 116(12):1001–1004

[17] Mullace M, Gorini E, Sbrocca M, Artesi L, Mevio N. Management of nasal septal perforation using silicone nasal septal button. Acta Otorhinolaryngol Ital. 2006; 26(4):216–218

[18] Federspil PA, Schneider M. [The custom made septal button]. Laryngorhinootologie. 2006; 85(5):323–325

[19] Artal S, Urpegui G, Alfonso C, Vallés H. Utilidad del botón septal y nivel de satisfacción obtenido en los pacientes con perforaciones del septum: Nuestra experiencia. Rev Otorrinolaringol Cir Cabeza Cuello. 2011; 71(2):145–154

[20] Illing E, Beer H, Webb C, Banhegyi G. Double septal button: a novel method of treating large anterior septal perforations. Clin Otolaryngol. 2013; 38(2):184–186

[21] Kim SW, Rhee CS. Nasal septal perforation repair: predictive factors and systematic review of the literature. Curr Opin Otolaryngol Head Neck Surg. 2012; 20(1):58–65

[22] Døsen LK, Haye R. Silicone button in nasal septal perforation. Long term observations. Rhinology. 2008; 46(4):324–327

Chapter 9
Free Grafts

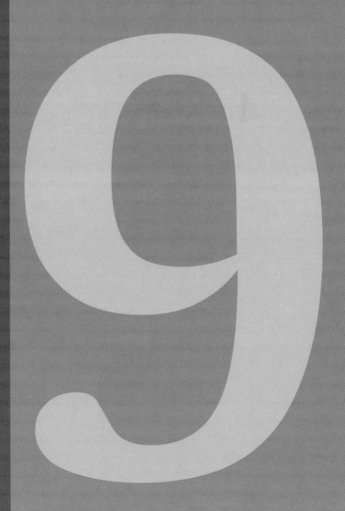

9 Free Grafts

Hesham A. K. A. Mansour

Summary

Free grafts can be used for repair of nasoseptal perforation either alone or as interposition grafts with advancement and/or rotational flaps. Interposition grafts are used to avoid excessive tension on the perforation closure suture line. The grafts serve as a template for mucosal and vascular regeneration during healing processes and prevent mucosal flaps from shrinking. Different grafts were used for this purpose including remnants of the septal cartilage or bone (vomer or perpendicular plate of ethmoid), auricular cartilage (conchal or tragal), acellular human dermal allograft, and temporalis fascia. The type of interposition graft does not affect the surgical outcome. Limited cases with alternative grafts are described (titanium membrane, bioactive glass, porcine small intestine submucosa).

The repair of nasoseptal perforation using free grafts alone or together with limited local flaps is discussed in this chapter. A technique using inferior turbinate free graft with no flaps is also discussed.

9.1 Indications

- Symptomatizing nasoseptal perforation not responding to conservative treatment.
- The size of perforation should be small to moderate.
- The inferior turbinate should be hypertrophic or normal but not atrophic or previously excised.
- Fibrosis of the septal mucosa or adherent mucosa (bipedicled or advancement flaps are difficult or impossible to elevate). In these cases this technique can be applied, as it does not imply elevation of much mucoperichondrium.

9.2 Surgical Steps

The repair is performed under general anesthesia using a closed endonasal endoscopic approach.

1. The mucoperichondrium on both sides and the inferior turbinate on the one side are infiltrated using 1/200,000 adrenaline with 1% lidocaine. A caudal septal incision (hemitransfixion) is made on the one side and subperichondrial dissection starts from anterior to posterior until the septal perforation is reached.
2. The edge of the perforation is entered and the dissection continues above and below the perforation.
3. At this point an endoscope (0 degree, 4 mm) is used. The edge of the perforation is incised superiorly, posteriorly, and inferiorly using a number 12 scalpel blade, and a tunnel is created by dissecting between the mucoperichondrium of both sides and between the mucoperichondrium and the septal cartilage on the one side (▶ Fig. 9.1).
4. A partial inferior turbinectomy is performed. The inferior turbinate graft is then flattened, taking care not to disturb its continuity (▶ Fig. 9.2).
5. Vicryl 4/0 sutures are used to fix the graft in place within the tunnel. The first stitch is made posteriorly by taking one bite about 5 mm posterior to the posterior edge of the perforation and the other bite into the graft. The graft is then approximated to the perforation and tucked into place as the stitch is tightened (▶ Fig. 9.3).
6. The graft is positioned between the mucoperichondrium of both sides and between the mucoperichondrium and the cartilage of the one side. The graft is fixed by more stitches positioned superiorly, inferiorly, and anteriorly (▶ Fig. 9.4, ▶ Fig. 9.5).
7. The anterior septal incision is then closed, and Silastic splints are applied to protect the graft and prevent adhesions. They are removed after 1 week (▶ Fig. 9.6).

This technique has the following advantages:
- The use of respiratory mucosa is physiologic, avoiding dryness that is the disadvantage when labial mucosa or skin grafts are being used.
- The ease of harvesting the graft and accessibility of the donor site.
- The graft is vascular and strong with easy handling, and leaving a part of turbinate bone adds to the support of the repaired area.
- There is limited mucoperichondrium elevation with no flap needed that means an easier procedure with no fear of further tear of the mucoperichondrium and mucoperiosteum or alteration of blood supply while elevating the flaps. This is of value especially if the septal mucosa is damaged because of excessive fibrosis or previous surgery.
- The use of this technique avoids tension on suture lines, which is the case when advancement or rotation flaps are being used.
- No need for a second-stage surgery to separate the flap from the donor site and no possibility of nasal obstruction secondary to bulky flaps.

Leaving a raw area on the one side is not a drawback as the septal mucosa was found to creep and cover the raw area within 3 to 5 weeks.[1,2,3]

Previously, similar technique using inferior turbinate composite graft was described in which the margin of the perforation was elevated using 20 G needle bent into

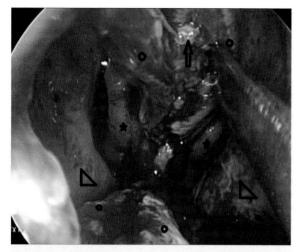

Fig. 9.1 Dissection between mucoperichondrium of both sides (small circles). Middle turbinates (stars). Inferior turbinates (arrowhead). Remnant of sepal cartilage (arrow).

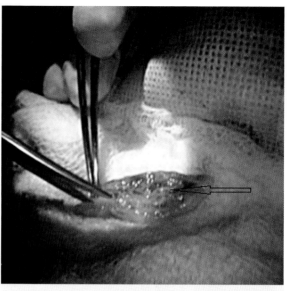

Fig. 9.2 Inferior turbinate graft is prepared and flattened with remnant of bone (arrow).

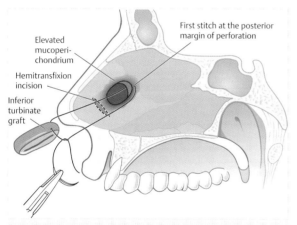

Fig. 9.3 A diagram showing the first stitch taken in the posterior margin of the perforation and the graft. As the suture is tightened, the graft is tucked in place.

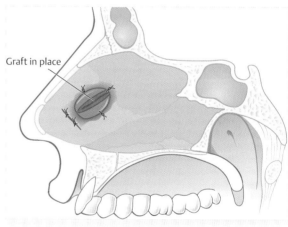

Fig. 9.4 A diagram showing the graft in place.

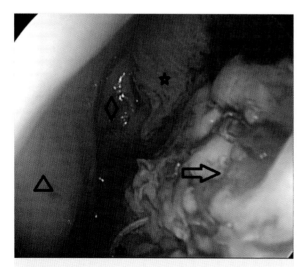

Fig. 9.5 The graft (arrow) is in place with sutures. Septum above and below (stars). Inferior turbinate (triangle). Middle turbinate (diamond).

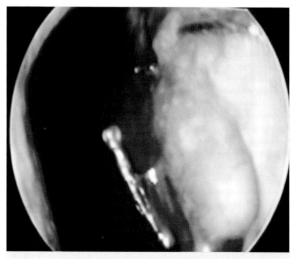

Fig. 9.6 One-week follow-up of the free graft.

appropriate angle for about 3 to 4 mm circumferentially. The latter technique was also performed in an endonasal endoscopic approach. The inferior turbinate graft was harvested such that two layers of turbinate mucosa and part of turbinate bone are included. This way of using the graft and the absence of septal incision are the differences between this technique and the one described previously. The same authors described another technique for larger perforations. A hemitransfixion incision was used and bipedicled flaps created and sutured with interposition of inferior turbinate graft.[4]

The same endonasal endoscopic approach and the steps described previously were applied using inferior turbinate graft with the addition of temporalis fascia to cover the raw surface of the inferior turbinate. This includes hemitransfixion incision and trimming the margin of perforation with a sickle knife in a preliminary study.[5]

Cassano described a technique using a combined endoscopic endonasal approach and a hemitransfixion incision. On the one side the advancement or rotation flap was created to close the defect. On the other side the mucoperichondrium was elevated and an inferior turbinate graft was applied.[6]

The mucosal regeneration technique was described using auricular conchal cartilage with perichondrium as a graft. While using open rhinoplasty approach, mucoperichondrium was elevated; the graft was shaped to fit the cartilage and bone defect and sutured to the remaining cartilage and bone without creation of advancement or rotational flaps. The mucosal defect was closed by secondary healing (over the graft was left for regeneration and reepithelization by the surrounding septal mucosa). This approach is similar to cartilage tympanoplasty waiting for remnant of the tympanic membrane to heal over the graft.[7,8] Although the mucosal regeneration technique was described using an open rhinoplasty approach, it would be possible to perform it endoscopically.

Conchal cartilage in combination with temporalis fascia is also described as a suitable graft in literature. Using this technique, the edge of the perforation is elevated by endonasal endoscopic approach and the graft is placed and fixed by bioabsorbable staples.[9]

Auricular conchal cartilage was also used as an interposition graft. The mucoperichondrium and mucoperiosteum were widely elevated up to the choana, nasal dome, and nasal floor. A vertical posterior and/or horizontal inferior relaxation incision can be added. The graft is kept in place by absorbable sutures to the residual septum.[10]

Autogenous septal graft (cartilage or bone) from behind the perforation was used as a graft. A pedicled local mucoperichondrial flap was created in the one side and the other side of the defect was left to heal secondarily.[11]

The residual septal cartilage or bone coated by quadriceps fascia was used for repair of septal perforation. In the same study middle turbinate free graft was also used in addition in larger perforation. Using endoscopic-assisted intranasal approach, the incision and dissection of the mucoperichondrium and mucoperiosteum is more or less the same as the steps described previously but with removal of crest of maxillary bone. No stitches were used.[12]

A technique using acellular dermis as a graft without the creation of local advancement or rotation flaps was described. A piece of medium-thickness acellular dermis was used to cover the defect by undermining the graft under the elevated mucoperichondrium. Bilateral Silastic splints were placed to hold the mucoperichondrium and the graft in place with one transseptal suture. No sutures were used to fix the graft and the defect was left for mucosalization by the surrounding mucoperichondrium.[13]

Acellular human dermal allograft was also used to repair septal perforation by endonasal endoscopic approach. A hemitransfixion incision is used to raise the mucoperichondrium on the one side and a rotational flap was created on the other side. The allograft was inserted between the cartilage and mucoperichondrium in underlay fashion on the opposite side.[14]

9.3 Case Example

A 45-year-old man with history of septal surgery 2 year ago was forwarded to our department. The patient presented nasal crusts with nasal obstruction and recurrent epistaxis. These symptoms did not improve on conservative treatment.

Nasal endoscopic examination demonstrated medium-sized septal perforation. No signs of past turbinal surgery were found and endoscopic approach with free graft was taken. Left hemitransfixion incision was made with dissection of the mucoperichondrium. Partial inferior turbinectomy was undertaken and the graft was fashioned. The inferior turbinate graft was flattened and tucked in place as described previously. The first stitch was made posteriorly by taking one bite about 5 mm posterior to the posterior edge of the perforation and the other bite into the graft. Silastic splints were left in place for 1 week. Daily nasal douches and ointments were recommended. It was noticed that raw surface of the graft is covered by mucosa within 8 weeks (▶ Fig. 9.7). Complete closure of the perforation was achieved with no further symptoms (▶ Fig. 9.8).

9.4 Complications

- Atrophy of nasal turbinate from where the graft is taken. This would lead to nasal dryness and crusts.
- Necrosis of the inferior turbinate graft after placement between mucoperichondrium on both sides. This possibility is high when the perforation is large and the graft has no enough peripheral blood supply to survive. This will lead to failure or residual perforation.
- Postoperative bleeding.
- Tear of the mucoperichondrium is rare and limited, as the technique does not include extensive elevation of flaps.

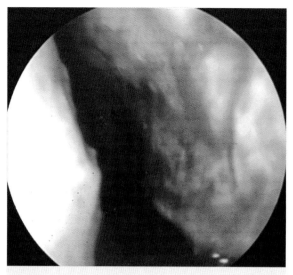

Fig. 9.7 Raw surface of the graft is covered by mucosa within 8 weeks.

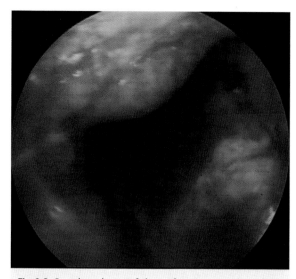

Fig. 9.8 Complete closure of the perforation was achieved 3 months after surgery.

9.5 Tips and Tricks

- Only partial turbinectomy should be performed leaving enough turbinate mucosa to avoid atrophic changes and crustation.
- The inferior turbinate graft is gently opened and flattened leaving part of the turbinate bone. This bone remnant will add to the strength of the graft.
- Only limited elevation of the mucoperichondrium is performed to accommodate the graft. This will avoid the tear of the mucoperichondrium, especially after previous attempt at repair.
- Cauterization of the remaining part of inferior turbinate that is highly vascular is necessary to avoid postoperative hemorrhage.
- Patients with large perforations are not candidates for this procedure. Even if a large graft is applied, partial or complete necrosis may be expected due to lack of enough peripheral blood supply.
- No technique is ideal for repair of all cases of nasoseptal perforation. The size and location of septal perforation, the condition of the mucoperichondrium, previous surgery, and pathologic condition of the nasal mucosa are all factors to determine the technique. In addition, the experience and the preference of the surgeon should be considered.

References

[1] Kim SW, Rhee CS. Nasal septal perforation repair: predictive factors and systematic review of the literature. Curr Opin Otolaryngol Head Neck Surg. 2012; 20(1):58–65

[2] Moon IJ, Kim SW, Han DH, et al. Predictive factors for the outcome of nasal septal perforation repair. Auris Nasus Larynx. 2011; 38(1):52–57

[3] Mansour HA. Repair of nasal septal perforation using inferior turbinate graft. J Laryngol Otol. 2011; 125(5):474–478

[4] Tastan E, Aydogan F, Aydin E, et al. Inferior turbinate composite graft for repair of nasal septal perforation. Am J Rhinol Allergy. 2012; 26(3):237–242

[5] Jeon EJ, Choi J, Lee JH, et al. The role of temporalis fascia for free mucosal graft survival in small nasal septal perforation repair. J Craniofac Surg. 2014; 25(2):e164–e166

[6] Cassano M. Endoscopic repair of nasal septal perforation with "slide and patch" technique. Otolaryngol Head Neck Surg. 2014; 151(1):176–178

[7] Yenigun A, Meric A, Verim A, Ozucer B, Yasar H, Ozkul MH. Septal perforation repair: mucosal regeneration technique. Eur Arch Otorhinolaryngol. 2012; 269(12):2505–2510

[8] Ozkul HM, Balikci HH, Karakas M, Bayram O, Bayram AA, Kara N. Repair of symptomatic nasoseptal perforations using mucosal regeneration technique with interpositional grafts. J Craniofac Surg. 2014; 25(1):98–102

[9] Kaya E, Cingi C, Olgun Y, Soken H, Pinarbasli Ö. Three layer interlocking: a novel technique for repairing a nasal septum perforation. Ann Otol Rhinol Laryngol. 2015; 124(3):212–215

[10] Giacomini PG, Ferraro S, Di Girolamo S, Ottaviani F. Large nasal septal perforation repair by closed endoscopically assisted approach. Ann Plast Surg. 2011; 66(6):633–636

[11] Li F, Liu Q, Yu H, Zhang Z. Pedicled local mucosal flap and autogenous graft for the closure of nasoseptal perforations. Acta Otolaryngol. 2011; 131(9):983–988

[12] Chen FH, Rui X, Deng J, Wen YH, Xu G, Shi JB. Endoscopic sandwich technique for moderate nasal septal perforations. Laryngoscope. 2012; 122(11):2367–2372

[13] Sharma A, Janus J, Diggelmann HR, Hamilton GS, III. Healing septal perforations by secondary intention using acellular dermis as a bioscaffold. Ann Otol Rhinol Laryngol. 2015; 124(6):425–429

[14] Chhabra N, Houser SM. Endonasal repair of septal perforations using a rotational mucosal flap and acellular dermal interposition graft. Int Forum Allergy Rhinol. 2012; 2(5):392–396

Chapter 10

Repair of Nasal Septal Perforation by Using Middle Turbinate Flap

10

10 Repair of Nasal Septal Perforation by Using Middle Turbinate Flap

Deniz Hanci, Huseyin Altun

Summary

Symptomatic nasal septal perforations often require surgical treatment. Repair of nasal septal perforation by using middle turbinate flap (monopedicled superiorly based bone included conchal flap) is a new unilateral middle turbinate mucosal flap technique. This chapter aims to describe the surgical technique of endoscope-assisted endonasal approach for the repair of septal perforations. The most appropriate middle turbinate for the surgical procedure bases according to its size, location, and computed tomographic (CT) scan.

10.1 Introduction

The incidence of nasal septal perforation is estimated at 1%.[1] In fact, the otolaryngologist has to identify the cause, which in most cases is either iatrogenic or idiopathic, to decide the need for surgery and select the most suitable surgical technique of those currently available, for the case under consideration.

Nasal septal perforations are complete defects of the mucosal and cartilaginous tissues of the nasal septum. These defects in the cartilaginous areas of the septum, with direct communication between the two nasal cavities, lead to impairment of the airflow, which is often accompanied by a wide variety of symptoms. Septal perforation may also be detected during routine medical examinations. Anterior and wide septal perforations are more symptomatic, whereas posterior perforations tend to be less symptomatic, due to humidification from the turbinates. While some of the perforations remain unnoticed by patients, in many cases of septal perforations patients suffer from recurrent epistaxis, nasal obstruction sensation, discharge, crusting, dryness, foreign-body sensation, headache, pain, and whistling. Nasal septal perforations differ widely in cause or origin. Symptoms in patients with nasal septal perforations are attributable to a physiologic disturbance in nasal airflow. Instead of the normal, parabolically shaped lamellar flow, the perforation creates turbulent flow, with a resultant decrease in the normal humidification process, resulting in crusting and desiccation of the affected area. Aggressive cauterization of nasal mucosa in epistaxis, self-induced trauma, external trauma, neoplasms (carcinoma, T-cell lymphomas), infectious diseases (e.g., syphilis, diphtheria, and tuberculosis), inflammatory diseases (sarcoidosis, Wegener's granulomatosis, systemic lupus erythematosus), inhalatory drug abuse, and iatrogenic perforations secondary to nasal septal surgery are possible etiologic factors.[2,3]

Management of nasal septal perforations initially requires medical treatment. Patients with significant intranasal crusting can be treated with nasal irrigation and a topical emollient. Dryness can be treated with topical nasal estrogenic spray.[4]

Symptomatic nasal septal perforations often require surgical treatment. Nasal irrigation and topical ointments do not improve the symptoms of the patients significantly. The use of septal obturator as a silicon grommet prosthesis is often not able to reduce the patient's symptoms and causes additional problems of foreign bodies in the nose. Resurfacing the defect with respiratory mucosa of nasal origin is the method of choice for closure of septal perforations. Surgical repair of the nasal septal perforation is indeed a difficult challenge for every rhinologist because of the high rate of reperforations. Many surgical approaches for repair of septal perforations have been reported in the literature[5] however, the available closure techniques are technically difficult and require experienced surgeons.

This chapter aims to describe and present our experiences with a new and simple surgical technique of endoscope-assisted endonasal approach for the repair of septal perforations.

The blood supply of the middle turbinate occurs by lateral branches of sphenopalatina artery and anterior ethmoidal artery.

10.2 Indications

Our technique suggested that the endonasal approach is adequate for surgical exposition of septal perforations, flap dissection, and suturing. The absence of external scars and morbidity on the donor site are advantages of this technique. The use of nasal endoscopy allows superior precision in all surgical steps by ensuring excellent exposure of the operative areas.

In our opinion, only techniques with nasal mucosal flaps achieve a normal nasal physiology because they use the normal respiratory epithelium for closure.[6] Our flaps, despite being monopedicled and often with wide dimensions, never showed a vascular suffering.

Numerous flap designs have been described in the literature. The main factor contributing to a high closure rate was the choice of a flap design, which suited the

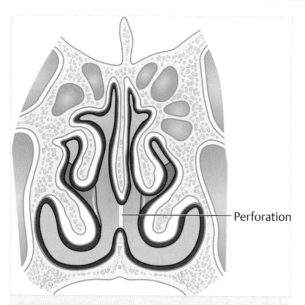

Fig. 10.1 Septal perforation in the middle of the septum.

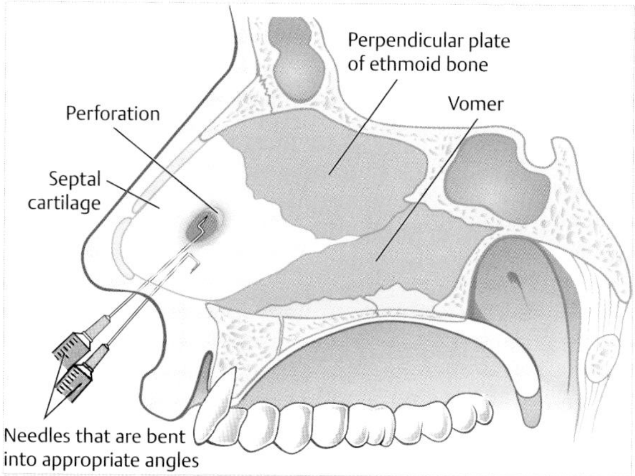

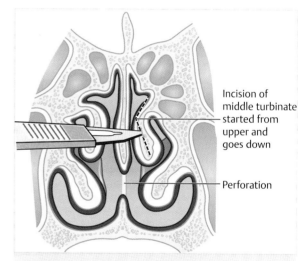

Fig. 10.2 Elevation of mucosal flaps by using needles that are bent into appropriate angles.

nasal septal perforation. This choice was dependent on perforation location (anterior or posterior) perforation size (the perforation size is inversely proportional to the amount of viable mucosal available to be used as a flap); ability to preserve the flap's vascular supply; and availability of viable intranasal tissue to be used as a flap.

A new flap with many advantages in comparison to the other surgical techniques is described in the present study. With this technique, the normal respiratory mucosa of the nose is used for the reconstruction of the anatomy and physiology of the nose. The mucosa of the turbinate shows a good vascularization, which promotes the healing process. An individual adaptation of the size of this mucosal bone flap to the size of the perforation is possible.

10.3 Surgical Steps

1. Under general anesthesia, the nasal septum and middle turbinate were injected with 1% lidocaine with 1:100,000 epinephrine solution to reduce intraoperative bleeding.
2. The nose was decongested using xylometazoline HCL (Otrivin) on cotton nasal pledgets. All patients received both intra- and postoperative antibiotics. After 5 minutes decongestion, both the nasal cavities were examined and septal perforation size was measured (▶ Fig. 10.1). Each surgical step was performed under endoscopic view.
3. The mucosa around the perforation was then incised circumferentially approximately 3 mm from its edge. Posterior margin of the perforation was easily elevated with a blade by using the tip of 20 G needle whereas angulated instruments were needed for the elevation

Fig. 10.3 Incision of middle turbinate is started from upper part of middle concha and goes down.

of mucosal flaps at the anterior, superior, and inferior margins of the perforation (▶ Fig. 10.2). The most appropriate middle turbinate was chosen for the surgical procedure, according to its size, location, and CT scan.
4. Chosen turbinate was then lateralized and dissected from the midline started from superior to inferior and anterior to posterior, and turbinate opened like leaf (▶ Fig. 10.3).
5. The conchal bone was removed circumferentially approximately 5 mm from its edge. This relaxing excision permits the creation of monopedicled conchal flap that includes superiorly conchal bone. The length of the flap was adapted to the size of the

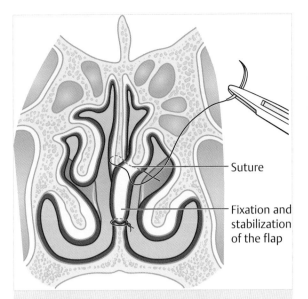

Fig. 10.4 Fixation and stabilization of the flap.

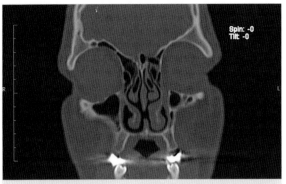

Fig. 10.5 A coronal computed sinus tomography shows septal perforation.

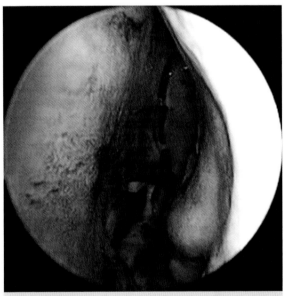

Fig. 10.6 An endoscopic view of septal perforation of one of the patients during surgery.

septal defect. It is more appropriate to harvest the graft slightly larger than the perforation size. The prepared conchal mucosal flap's anterior, posterior, and inferior parts were positioned between muco-perichondrial flap and septal cartilage in inferior, posterior, and anterior parts. The flap was then sutured to the septal mucosa of the anterior, posterior, and inferior margins of the perforation, with a reabsorbable suture (5–0 polyglycolic acid) (▶ Fig. 10.4). Silastic splints were subsequently placed bilaterally. The nasal splints were removed after 10 days postoperatively in the clinic. Saline nasal drops and antibiotic cream were prescribed to keep the nose moist and clean during the post-operative 30 days period. Endoscopic control of the surgical site was made in this period. After 2 months, flap pedicles in all patients were cut by a scissors under local anesthesia. Bipolar cauterization was used to control bleeding. ▶ Table 10.1 presents some points of difficulty and technical solutions.

Table 10.1 Points of difficulty and technical solutions

Adaptation of the length of the flap to the size of septal defect	Harvest the graft slightly larger than the perforation size
Choosing appropriate middle turbinate	Use computed tomography
Desepitalization of the anterior part of the perforation	Use curved needle
Crusting of the mucosa	Use ointment and use silicon nasal splint for 10 days

10.4 Case Examples

10.4.1 Case 1

A 40-year-old man presented with history of difficulty in breathing and allergic rhinitis. He had septoplasty and turbinoplasty surgery 3 years ago. He had complained about rhinorrhea, crusting, and epistaxis. Nasal endoscopic examination revealed septal perforation about 1.5 cm (length). The CT scan showed septal perforation in the midportion of the septum, bilateral concha bullosa, and left inferior conchal hypertrophy (▶ Fig. 10.5). The patient was scheduled for endoscopic repair of septal perforation with middle turbinate flap. Pre- and post-operative endoscopic views of the septum were provided (▶ Fig. 10.6, ▶ Fig. 10.7).

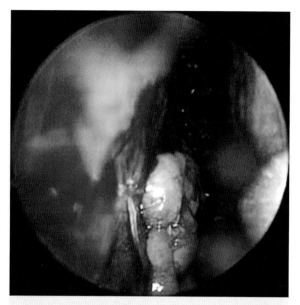

Fig. 10.7 An endoscopic view of the closed septal perforation with conchal flap in the end of the surgery.

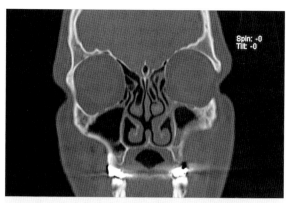

Fig. 10.8 A coronal computed sinus tomography shows septal perforation.

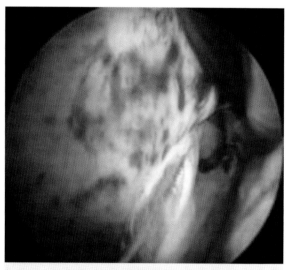

Fig. 10.9 An endoscopic view of septal perforation of one of the patients during surgery.

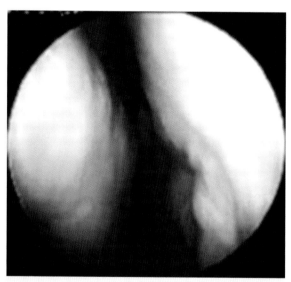

Fig. 10.10 An endoscopic view of the closed septal perforation with conchal flap after 3 months.

10.4.2 Case 2

A 38-year-old woman presented with history of nasal stuffiness and sinusitis. The patient had septoplasty and conchal radiofrequency surgery 6 years ago. She had complained about crusting and epistaxis. Nasal endoscopic examination revealed septal perforation about 1 cm (length) with crusting. The CT scan showed septal perforation in the midportion of the septum and conchal hypertrophy (▶ Fig. 10.8). The patient was scheduled for endoscopic repair of septal perforation with middle turbinate flap. Pre- and postoperative endoscopic views of the septum were provided (▶ Fig. 10.9, ▶ Fig. 10.10).

10.5 Tips and Tricks

- This method is not usable for the perforation of anterior part of the septum.
- Use angulated instrument for desepitalization mucosa around the perforation.
- Harvest the graft larger than the perforation size.
- CT is useful to choose this method for the repairs of the perforation.

References

[1] Ohlsén L. Closure of nasal septal perforation with a cutaneous flap and a perichondrocutaneous graft. Ann Plast Surg. 1988; 21(3):276–288

[2] Lanier B, Kai G, Marple B, Wall GM. Pathophysiology and progression of nasal septal perforation. Ann Allergy Asthma Immunol. 2007; 99 (6):473–479, quiz 480–481, 521

[3] Døsen LK, Haye R. Nasal septal perforation 1981–2005: changes in etiology, gender and size. BMC Ear Nose Throat Disord. 2007; 7:1–4

[4] Batniji RK, Chmiel JF. Septal perforations: medical aspects. E- medicine. http://www.emedicine.com/ent/topic704.htm. Accessed November 10, 2016

[5] Goh AY, Hussain SS. Different surgical treatments for nasal septal perforation and their outcomes. J Laryngol Otol. 2007; 121(5):419–426

[6] Kridel RWH. Considerations in the etiology, treatment, and repair of septal perforations. Facial Plast Surg Clin North Am. 2004; 12(4): 435–450, vi

Chapter 11
Inferior Turbinate Flap

11 Inferior Turbinate Flap

Cristobal Langdon, Isam Alobid

Summary

There are many surgical techniques available for surgical repair of nasal septal perforations (NSPs), but the evidence shows that no single technique is recognized as being consistently reliable. The inferior turbinate flap (ITF) for repair of NSPs of moderate size is a relatively simple technique that offers a success rate comparable to most techniques. The key advantages of the ITF include abundant vascularity, wide arc of rotation, possibility to use a combined skeletal and epithelial support, and ease of harvesting and insertion. Even more, any endoscopic surgeon can master the technique, and it can be one more substitute solution to a difficult problem.

11.1 Indications

- Medium (1–2 cm) and/or large (> 2 cm) size NSPs
- NSP without osteocartilaginous support
- Rescue flap for NSP

11.2 Contraindications

- In any patient who has undergone sphenopalatine artery or anterior ethmoidal artery ligation on the ipsilateral side.
- Previous inferior turbinectomy or inferior turbinate (IT) surgery may reduce the flap's pliability, limit its ability to mold to the shape of the defect, and may also compromise its blood supply.

11.3 Anatomy

The IT bone develops from a cartilage ossification center during the fifth intrauterine month. At the core of the IT is its central osseous layer of nonhomogeneous, cancellous, sponge-like bone made of interwoven bony trabeculae separated by a labyrinth of interconnecting spaces containing fatty tissue and blood vessels. The histology of the IT is comprises an epithelial mucosal layer overlying a basement membrane, an osseous layer, and an intervening lamina propria. The medial aspect of the mucosal layer is thicker and has more surface area than the lateral mucosa of the turbinate.[1]

IT is vascularized by the posterolateral nasal artery (PLNA) (▶ Fig. 11.1). The PLNA descends vertically and slightly forward over the vertical apophysis of the palatine bone and enters the IT on the superior aspect of its lateral attachment between 1.0 and 1.5 cm from its posterior insertion. In 15% of cases the IT may receive supplementary irrigation from the palatine artery branches of the descending palatine artery.[2] Wu et al[3] studied the vascular anatomy of the IT in 11 cadavers. They observed that mean outer diameter of the PLNA is 1.10 ± 0.11 mm (range: 0.82–1.30); and it enters the IT on the superior aspect of its lateral attachment, 1.0 to 1.5 cm from its posterior tip; and divides in 2.50 ± 0.52 (range: 2–3) arteries as part of IT circulation. After the division the arteries enter a bony canal; one branch remains high and lateral while the other runs in a lower and more medial position. Both remain in bony canals or are closely applied to the bone for much of the length of the turbinate. The lower (medial) branch gives off branches that pierce the bone of the interior turbinate in its anterior part and form a

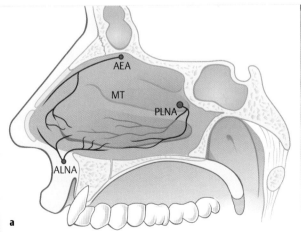

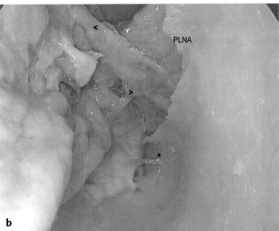

Fig. 11.1 (a) Scheme of the inferior turbinate vascularization. AEA, anterior ethmoidal artery; ANLA, anterior lateral nasal artery (branch of the facial artery); MT, middle turbinate; PLNA, posterior lateral nasal artery. (b) Endoscopic photograph of the inferior turbinate arteries. PLNA, posterior lateral nasal artery; <, superior lateral inferior turbinate artery; >, inferior medial inferior turbinate artery; *, branch of the descending palatine artery to the inferior turbinate.

regular pattern of alternating superior and inferior branches at right angles to the main artery. As the arteries run anteriorly, they increase in size, suggesting that there is a significant additional blood flow from anteriorly. These blood supplies are from an anastomosis with the anterior ethmoidal artery and the lateral nasal artery, which is a branch of the facial artery.

The ITF presents an excellent anteroposterior distance but lacks of a wide width. Gras-Cabrerizo et al[4] studied four cadaveric specimens and showed an anteroposterior distance range between 4.2 and 5 cm, with a width range between 1.2 and 1.4 cm. Amit et al[5] obtained similar results with a mean length and width of 4.8 and 1.8 cm, respectively, in 11 cadaver specimens. Harvey et al[6] obtained a similar length (5.4 cm), but with greater width (2.2 cm) extending its dissection to the inferior meatus and/or fossa floor.

11.4 Surgical Steps

11.4.1 Sinonasal Cavity Preparation

Cottonoids impregnated with a solution of 1:10,000 epinephrine are placed in the nasal cavity bilaterally during the surgical setup. At the beginning of surgery, the sites corresponding to the planned incisions are injected with lidocaine 1% with epinephrine 1:100,000. One must avoid injecting the area adjacent to the flap's vascular pedicle (i.e., it causes vasospasm of the pedicle potentially impairing its viability) and the interior turbinate (i.e., it may be equivalent to an intravascular injection).

11.4.2 Posteriorly Based Inferior Turbinate Flap: Surgical Technique

1. The nasal cavity is decongested and prepared as previously described.
2. The IT can be gently medialized to better visualize its medial surface and the mucosa from the inferior meatus, and then subsequently laterally fractured to gain access to the lateral nasal wall.
3. An uncinectomy allows the identification of the natural ostium of the maxillary sinus and the posterior portion of the IT. In some cases enlargement of the maxillary sinus ostium posteriorly allows a better exposure of the PLNA and eases the preservation of the pedicle (▶ Fig. 11.2).
4. Elevate the mucosa from the anterior aspect of the ascending process of the palatine bone in a submucoperiosteal plane and proceed posteriorly to identify the crista ethmoidalis, sphenopalatine foramen, and sphenopalatine artery and its terminal branches. The sphenopalatine foramen is identified superior to the posterior IT, posterior to the basal lamellae of the middle turbinate. The pedicle blood supply to the IT can sometimes be visualized as pulsating. There is

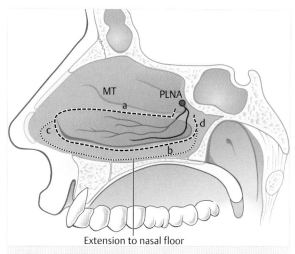

Fig. 11.2 Posteriorly based inferior turbinate flap (pITF). Schematic drawing showing the incision to raise a pITF. Care must be taken when performing the posterior incision as the PLNA runs just anteriorly to the place where the posterior incision is made. MT, middle turbinate; PLNA, posterior lateral nasal artery; a, superior incision; b, inferior incision; c, anterior incision; d posterior incision.

significant anatomical variation of the sphenopalatine artery branches and, accordingly, the sphenopalatine foramen or foramina. In fact, the PLNA may extend anterior to the posterior wall of the maxillary antrum.[7,8] Recognizing this anatomic variation during the maxillary antrostomy and mucoperiosteal elevation is vital to avoiding injury to the vascular pedicle.

5. Define the superior and inferior limits of the flap.
   a) Make a posterior to anterior incision along the superior sagittal plane of the IT (*superior incision*).
   b) Then make an inferior sagittal incision along the inferior meatus (*inferior incision*); in some cases one can extend the flap to the inferior meatus and nasal floor.
6. A vertical incision at the head of the IT then connects the two incisions (*anterior incision*). This incision is in S-shape, starting from the superior incision and sloping around the contour of the head of the IT and onto the inferior meatus. Care should be taken to avoid disrupting the valve of Hasner.
7. Use a periosteal elevator (freer dissector or Cottle elevator) to raise the mucoperiosteum off the IT from anterior to posterior both medial and lateral to the IT bone. The donor site is left open and allowed to heal, which is frequently the case after partial turbinectomy.
8. After harvesting the flap, margins of the perforation are easily elevated and/or rimmed with a 12-blade or a phaco blade. The two mucosal layers surrounding the perforation edges are separated from each other at least 3 to 4 mm in width circumferentially.

9. Finally the edges are sutured with absorbable suture (i.e., 2–0 Vicryl). Usually anterior, middle, and posterior sutures are placed to achieve complete closure. Sometimes the posterior sutures are difficult to place and they are reserve for the second surgery when the pedicle is detached from the lateral wall.

10. Second stage: After 6 weeks to 6 months, the pedicle is detached from the lateral nasal wall; bipolar cautery is used for hemostasis. The pedicle is transacted and the excess pedicle is discarded. At 3 weeks after surgery, the contralateral side of the flap has usually reepithelialized. Patients are instructed to keep the sides moist with nasal saline spray during the 3-week period.

11.4.3 Anteriorly Based Inferior Turbinate Flap

1. Repeat steps (1–5) of the PITF.
2. Because the pedicle of this flap is based anteriorly, care is taken not to injure the branches of the AEA, which passes anterior to the agger nasi. These branches arc below the nasal bone and spine of the frontal bone in a C-shaped loop before entering the IT.
3. Cauterization of the PLNA with bipolar/monopolar cautery or clips can be used.
4. Prolong the *posterior incision* through the tail of the IT in front of the eustachian tube and below to the inferior meatus. This step is crucial to free the posterior margin of the flap.
5. The entire portion of the IT is usually harvested.

6. Next, the mucoperiosteum covering the turbinate is elevated in an anterior to posterior direction with the use of a Cottle elevator and endoscopic scissors. The flap includes the entire mucosa of the IT, and it is detached from its inferior and lateral attachments (▶ Fig. 11.3).
7. Finally the AITF is based anteriorly and vascularized by the AEA and branches of the anterolateral nasal artery (ALNA) (▶ Fig. 11.4).
8. After harvesting the flap, margins of the perforation are easily elevated and/or rimmed with a 12-blade or a phaco blade. The two mucosal layers surrounding the perforation edges are separated from each other at least 3 to 4 mm in width circumferentially.
9. Finally the edges are sutured with absorbable suture (i.e., 2–0 Vicryl). Usually anterior, middle, and posterior sutures are placed to achieve complete closure. Sometimes the posterior sutures are difficult to place and they are reserve for the second surgery when the pedicle is detached from the lateral wall.
10. After 6 weeks to 6 months, the pedicle is detached from the lateral nasal wall; bipolar cautery is used for hemostasis. The pedicle is transacted and the excess pedicle is discarded. At 3 weeks after surgery, the contralateral side of the flap has usually reepithelialized. Patients are instructed to keep the sides moist with nasal saline spray during the 3-week period.

11.4.4 Postoperative Care

Nasal packing is removed in 48 to 72 hours taking care not to displace the Silastic sheets. Nasal saline douches are indicated three times, with at least 100 cc of saline per fossa. Topic vitamin A ointment for nasal vestibule is recommended twice a day; this helps hydrate and maintain a humid cavity after surgery. It is of utmost

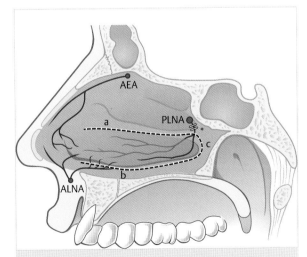

Fig. 11.3 Anteriorly based inferior turbinate flap (aITF). Schematic drawing showing the incision to raise an aITF. AEA, anterior ethmoidal artery; ANLA, anterior lateral nasal artery (branch of the facial artery); PLNA, posterior lateral nasal artery; a, superior incision; b, inferior incision; c, posterior incision; *, clipping or cauterization of PLNA.

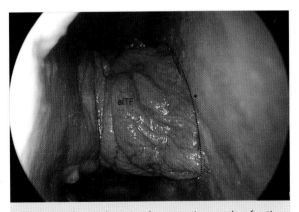

Fig. 11.4 Cadaveric dissection demonstrating septal perforation reconstruction by the anteriorly based inferior turbinate flap (aITF). *, anterior margin of the septal perforation completely closed by the flap.

importance to visit the patient on a weekly-based schedule for the first month. Thorough aspiration of nasal secretions and removal of crusts avoiding tension over the flap are equally important. Remove the Silastic sheets between 2 to 3 weeks postoperatively. The donor surface of the flap heals by secondary intention producing crusting during the healing process.[9,10]

11.5 Case Example

A 65-year-old man with diagnosis of sleep obstructive breathing disorder under treatment with continuous positive airway pressure (CPAP) presented with crusting, dryness, and nasal obstruction. Examination revealed a 2.5-cm NSP (▶ Fig. 11.5). He had a surgical history of septoplasty.

The computed tomographic (CT) scan showed an anterior septal defect with scare osteocartilaginous support (▶ Fig. 11.6). Both ITs where intact and no sign of sinus opacification was shown.

The patient was scheduled for endonasal endoscopic closure of NSP with a posteriorly based ITF. After 3 months of the surgery, he had a magnetic resonance imaging (MRI) of the head indicated by the neurologist In that image one can observe the perfect integration of the anterior portion of the ITF to the nasal septum (▶ Fig. 11.7). Finally 6 months after the surgery, the patient was scheduled for endonasal endoscopic surgery to release the posterior attachment of the ITF and close the posterior portion of the septal defect (▶ Fig. 11.8).

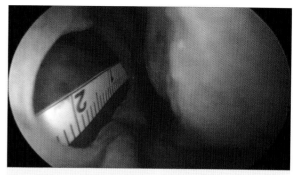

Fig. 11.5 Endoscopic view (0-degree lens), left nasal cavity. Septal perforation of 2.5 cm anteroposteriorly.

11.6 Discussion

Local nasal septal flaps have been the most common surgical treatments for NSP up till now.[9,11,12] Successful repair of septal perforation depends on numerous factors. The size of the perforation is an important predictor of successful closure,[13] so larger septal perforations are more difficult to close surgically. Vertical size of a perforation is more important because the advancement of the mucoperichondrial edges from the floor of the nose to the dorsum causes a greater tension. Kim and Rhee[14] performed a systematic review to evaluate predictive factor for closure success. They observed that the size of perforation was the most significant factor for complete closure. Surgical failure occurred more frequently in patients with large perforation (> 2 cm) than in those with small

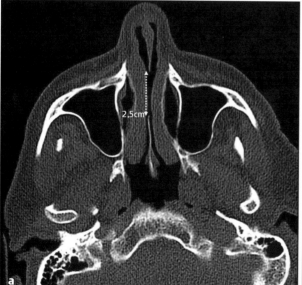
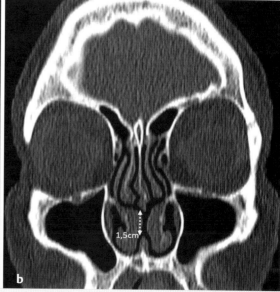

Fig. 11.6 (a) CT scan, axial view. White arrow shows the anteroposterior extension of the septal perforation. No sinus opacification are shown; inferior turbinates are preserve and without pathology. (b) CT scan, coronal view. White arrow shows the extension height of the septal perforation.

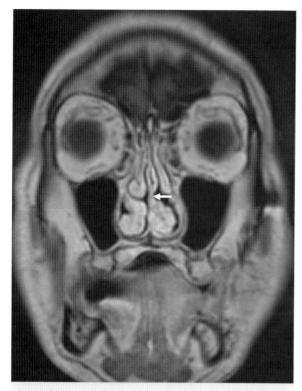

Fig. 11.7 Magnetic resonance imaging, coronal plane. White arrow shows the complete closure of the anterior portion of the septal perforation by the inferior turbinate flap.

to moderate perforation (< 2 cm). Moreover, the bilateral coverage over the perforation with vascularized mucosal flap eased a complete closure.

In 1980 Masing et al[15] introduced the ITF for closure of septal perforation. They reported a promising rate of nearly 80% of complete closure. Eight years later Vuyk and Versluis,[16] using a variation of the technique of Masing et al, were able to completely close only 30% of their perforations. Similar results were reported by Murakami et al.[17] They were able to close only three of the eight NSPs they repaired (38%), and two other patients had residual pinpoint perforations but were symptom free. Friedman et al,[9] after a minimum of 18 months' followup, successfully closed 70% of the NSPs they treated. More recently Tastan et al[18] in 27 patients, using an ITF alone or in combination with bipedicled mucosal advancement flap, achieved a complete closure of the perforation in 24 (88.8%) of 27 patients, and incomplete closure was observed only in 2 patients with medium-sized perforation and 1 patient with large perforation.

The ITF technique has the advantage of bringing tissue with a nourishing vascular supply into the septal defect, as the ITs have a double vascularization coming from both a descending branch of the sphenopalatine artery posteriorly and a branch of the facial artery adjacent to the piriform aperture anteriorly. A second advantage of this flap is the volume of tissue that is available for transfer. Murakami et al[17] showed in a small cadaver study that, on average, the IT mucosa has a surface area of nearly 5 cm². The main drawback to the ITF is the requirement of a second stage to free the flap from the lateral nasal wall. Between both stages patients usually complain about nasal obstruction, as the abundance of tissue that makes it a reliable flap may have enough bulk to cause partial

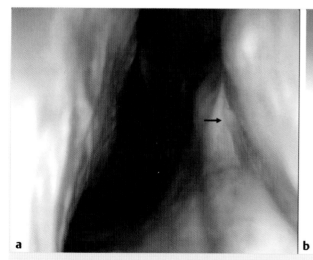

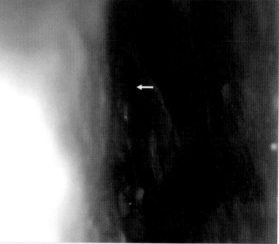

Fig. 11.8 (a) Right nasal fossa, posterior portion of the nasal fossa. Black arrow indicates the close posterior border of the perforation. (b) Left nasal fossa, anterior portion of nasal fossa. White arrow indicates the integrated and close anterior border of the perforation by the inferior turbinate flap. Although the flap is bulky, the patient did not complain about the nasal breathing, so no reduction in the flap was necessary.

Table 11.1 Complications and technical solutions

Complications	Technical solution
Bleeding from the PLNA or some inferior turbinate artery while harvesting the flap	Gentle harvest of the flap in a subperiosteal manner to leave the arteries inside the mucoperiosteal flap.
Preservation of the PLNA	Stay 1 cm anteriorly to the posterior insertion of the inferior turbinate.
Preservation of the AEA branches	Stay 1 cm posteriorly to the anterior insertion of the inferior turbinate.
Infection of the denuded inferior turbinate bone remnant	Remove all denuded bone and/or thorough postoperative care can prevent infection.
Reperforation of the nasal septum	Overcorrect the nasal defect at flap that is at least 20–30% bigger than the defect as the flap will shrink during the healing process.
Bulky flap that results in nasal obstruction	One can trim the bulky flap with a microdebrider. Use of radiofrequency to shrink the inferior turbinate tissue.
Nasal synechia	Thorough postoperative care removing all the fibrin will prevent synechia.

Abbreviations: AEA, anterior ethmoidal artery; PLNA, posterior lateral nasal artery.

obstruction of the airway. Assessment of the appropriate flap volume is important in preventing this complication. Another disadvantage is that one surface is not epithelialized and must heal by secondary ingrowth of epithelium. Finally, endoscopic closure of septal perforation by means of ITFs requires a considerable learning curve, and increased familiarity with these flaps improves flap survival and treatment outcome.

11.7 Conclusion

The ITF technique provides a nontension closure in perforations located anteriorly and medially, or previous unsuccessful surgical repair. The abundance of IT tissue makes it a robust and reliable flap, especially in cases where no osteocartilaginous support is available. However, at the same time, it also has enough bulk to cause partial obstruction of the airway so patients must return for a second operation to release the pedicle of the IT.

11.8 Complications

See ▶ Table 11.1.

11.9 Tips and Tricks

- Always assess for the osteocartilaginous support surrounding the nasal perforation. If there is no support, one can use the IT bone as support.
- Harvest of the flap should always be subperiosteally to avoid damaging the arterial pedicles.
- Stay at least 1 cm anteriorly to the posterior insertion of the IT to avoid damaging the PLNA.
- Rim the perforation in the final step of the surgery to avoid bleedings during the harvest of the flap.

References

References in bold are recommended readings.

[1] Berger G, Balum-Azim M, Ophir D. The normal inferior turbinate: histomorphometric analysis and clinical implications. Laryngoscope. 2003; 113(7):1192–1198

[2] Orhan M, Midilli R, Gode S, Saylam CY, Karci B. Blood supply of the inferior turbinate and its clinical applications. Clin Anat. 2010; 23(7): 770–776

[3] Wu P, Li Z, Liu C, Ouyang J, Zhong S. The posterior pedicled inferior turbinate-nasoseptal flap: a potential combined flap for skull base reconstruction. Surg Radiol Anat. 2015

[4] Gras-Cabrerizo JR, Ademá-Alcover JM, Gras-Albert JR, et al. Anatomical and surgical study of the sphenopalatine artery branches. Eur Arch Otorhinolaryngol. 2014; 271(7):1947–1951

[5] Amit M, Cohen J, Koren I, Gil Z. Cadaveric study for skull base reconstruction using anteriorly based inferior turbinate flap. Laryngoscope. 2013; 123(12):2940–2944

[6] Harvey RJ, Sheahan PO, Schlosser RJ. Inferior turbinate pedicle flap for endoscopic skull base defect repair. Am J Rhinol Allergy. 2009; 23 (5):522–526

[7] Schwartzbauer HR, Shete M, Tami TA. Endoscopic anatomy of the sphenopalatine and posterior nasal arteries: implications for the endoscopic management of epistaxis. Am J Rhinol. 2003; 17(1):63–66

[8] Chiu T. A study of the maxillary and sphenopalatine arteries in the pterygopalatine fossa and at the sphenopalatine foramen. Rhinology. 2009; 47(3):264–270

[9] **Friedman M, Ibrahim H, Ramakrishnan V. Inferior turbinate flap for repair of nasal septal perforation. Laryngoscope. 2003; 113(8): 1425–1428**

[10] Alobid I, Mason E, Solares CA, et al. Pedicled lateral nasal wall flap for the reconstruction of the nasal septum perforation. A radio-anatomical study. Rhinology. 2015; 53(3):235–241

[11] **Teymoortash A, Hoch S, Eivazi B, Werner JA. Experiences with a new surgical technique for closure of large perforations of the nasal septum in 55 patients. Am J Rhinol Allergy. 2011; 25(3):193–197**

[12] Islam A, Celik H, Felek SA, Demirci M. Repair of nasal septal perforation with "cross-stealing" technique. Am J Rhinol Allergy. 2009; 23 (2):225–228

[13] André RF, Lohuis PJ, Vuyk HD. Nasal septum perforation repair using differently designed, bilateral intranasal flaps, with nonopposing suture lines. J Plast Reconstr Aesthet Surg. 2006; 59(8): 829–834

[14] Kim SW, Rhee CS. Nasal septal perforation repair: predictive factors and systematic review of the literature. Curr Opin Otolaryngol Head Neck Surg. 2012; 20(1):58–65

[15] Masing H, Gammert C, Jaumann MP. [Our concept concerning treatment of septal perforations (author's transl)]. Laryngol Rhinol Otol (Stuttg). 1980; 59(1):50–56

[16] Vuyk HD, Versluis RJ. The inferior turbinate flap for closure of septal perforations. Clin Otolaryngol Allied Sci. 1988; 13(1):53–57

[17] Murakami CS, Kriet JD, Ierokomos AP. Nasal reconstruction using the inferior turbinate mucosal flap. Arch Facial Plast Surg. 1999; 1(2):97–100

[18] Tastan E, Aydogan F, Aydin E, et al. Inferior turbinate composite graft for repair of nasal septal perforation. Am J Rhinol Allergy. 2012; 26 (3):237–242

Chapter 12
Lateral Nasal Wall Flap

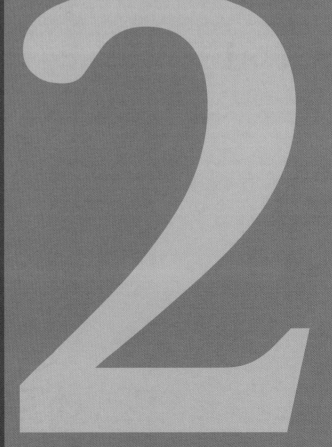

12 Lateral Nasal Wall Flap

Cristobal Langdon, Mauricio López-Chacón, Arturo Cordero Castillo, Alfonso Santamaría, Paula Mackers, Isam Alobid

Summary

Recently, a novel technique based on the use of pedicle lateral nasal wall (PLNW) flaps, either anterior (APLNW) or posterior (PPLNW), has proven to be a reliable and versatile reconstructive option for extensive defects of the skull base. Based on the later evidence, a PLNW flap may serve as an alternative procedure to reconstruct large nasal septum defects. The lateral nasal wall receives blood supply from a multiple anterior, posterior, and superior arterial branches, although its main arterial trunk arises posteriorly from the posterior lateral nasal artery (a branch of the sphenopalatine artery). The lateral alar artery (branch of the facial artery) and anterior ethmoidal artery supply the anterior and superior areas of the APLNW flap. These blood supplies may allow an anteriorly or posteriorly PLNW flap design to close septal perforations.

12.1 Indications

- Medium (1–2 cm) and/or large (> 2 cm) size nasal septal perforations
- Nasal septal perforation without osteocartilaginous support
- Rescue flap for nasal septal reperforation

12.2 Contraindications

- History of cauterization or embolization of sphenopalatine artery
- History of cauterization of anterior ethmoidal artery
- History of dacryocystorhinostomy on the ipsilateral side of the flap

12.3 Anatomy

Understanding the vascular anatomy of the lateral nasal wall is crucial for harvesting the PLNW.[1,2] The useful area of mucosa of the PLNW (▶ Fig. 12.1a, b) covers superiorly from the axilla of the middle turbinate, then goes inferiorly up to the piriform aperture until the floor of the nose, and inferiorly it goes to the posterior insertion of the inferior turbinate. Finally, a superior sagittal plane limits it extension at the level of the lateral wall of the maxillary sinus till the perpendicular plate of the palatine bone where the posterolateral nasal artery (PLNA) is found. Depending on the defect, one can use anteriorly or posteriorly based flaps. The anteriorly based flaps will receive most of its blood supply from the anterior ethmoidal artery branch of the ophthalmic artery and anterior-lateral nasal artery (ALNA) branch of the facial artery. Posteriorly based flap are based on the branches of the sphenopalatine artery, mainly from the PLNA (▶ Fig. 12.2). In the mucosa of the lateral nasal wall, the PLNA runs anteroinferiorly over the perpendicular plate of the palatine bone and gives branches to the middle

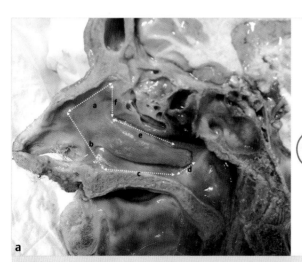
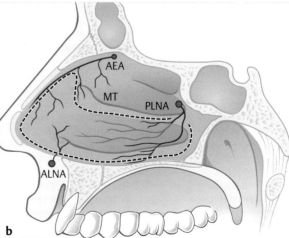

Fig. 12.1 (a) Incision of the lateral nasal wall flap. Right lateral nasal wall, cadaveric preparation. (a) anterosuperior incision; (b) anterior incision; (c) inferior incision; (d) posterior incision; (e) fontanelle incision; (f) maxillary line incision. (b) Schematic drawing of right posterior pedicle lateral wall flap. AEA, anterior ethmoidal artery; ALNA, anterior-lateral nasal artery; MT, middle turbinate; PLNA, posterior-lateral nasal artery; dotted line, surface of the right posterior pedicle lateral wall flap.

and inferior turbinates and fontanelle. Lee et al[3] studied 50 cadaveric specimens and observed that the PLNA ran downward on the perpendicular plate of the palatine bone and then coursed a little posterior to the posterior wall of the maxillary sinus in 42% and anterior to the posterior wall in 18%. Wu et al[4] studied the vascular anatomy of the PLNA in 11 cadavers. They observed that the PLNA mean outer diameter is 1.10 ± 0.11 (range: 0.82–1.30) mm and enters the inferior turbinate on the superior aspect of its lateral attachment, 1 to 1.5 cm from its posterior tip, and divides in 2.50 ± 0.52 (range: 2–3) arteries as part of inferior turbinate circulation.

Regarding the anatomy of the flap, Alobid et al[5] conducted a study on 40 de-identified computed tomographic (CT) angiographies and 20 hemicranial cadaver specimens to correlate the area and length of the PLNW flap with the nasal septum in order to plan surgery for septal perforation. On CT angiographies they demonstrated an average PLNW flap area of 10.80 ± 1.13 cm^2, with a septal area (22.54 ± 21.32 cm^2) that was significantly larger than the total PLNW flap area (14.59 ± 1.21 cm^2). The average length of the flap was 5.58 ± 0.39 cm, whereas the septum was 6.66 ± 0.42 cm; therefore, the PLNW flap is insufficient to reconstruct the entire septum. On the cadaver study, they showed that the length of the PLNW flap was 5.28 ± 0.40 cm. These results demonstrate that measurements obtained from CT scans are reliable data and similar to those found in the radiologic study, and one can repair at least 80% defect with a PLNW flap. Regarding anteriorly based flap for septal perforation, there is no evidence available, and even though it is feasible, the managing of the flap itself is difficult and it has a limited range of movement.

12.4 Surgical Steps

12.4.1 Sinonasal Cavity Preparation

Cottonoids impregnated with a solution of 1:10,000 epinephrine are placed in the nasal cavity bilaterally during the surgical setup. At the beginning of surgery, the sites corresponding to the planned incisions are injected with lidocaine 1% with epinephrine 1:100,000. One must avoid injecting the area adjacent to the flap's vascular pedicle (i.e., it causes vasospasm of the pedicle potentially impairing its viability) and the inferior turbinate (i.e., it may be equivalent to an intravascular injection).

12.4.2 Detailed Surgical Technique

- The PLNW flap is designed according to the size and shape of the defect. The floor and lateral nasal wall is infiltrated with a solution of bupivacaine (0.25%) containing epinephrine (1:100,000).
- Incisions can be made with a monopolar electrocautery using an extended, insulated, needle tip (Valley Lab, Boulder, Colorado) or an extended Colorado tip (Stryker Corporation, Kalamazoo, Michigan). Alternatively, the mucoperiosteum can be incised with a contact laser, Cottle elevator, or any other sharp instrument of preference.
- Start with an incision following the maxillary line (corresponded intranasally to the junction of the uncinate and the frontal process of the maxillary bone).
- Then continue with an anterosuperior incision (▶ Fig. 12.3) that runs anterior to the axilla of the middle turbinate downward down to the piriform aperture in front of the head of the inferior turbinate.

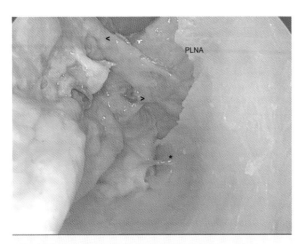

Fig. 12.2 Endoscopic photograph of the inferior turbinate arteries. PLNA, posterior lateral nasal artery; <, superior lateral inferior turbinate artery; >, inferior medial inferior turbinate artery; *, branch of the descending palatine artery to the inferior turbinate.

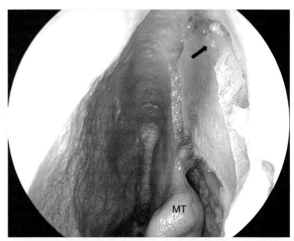

Fig. 12.3 Endoscopic view, 45-degree scope. Left lateral nasal wall anterosuperior incision (black arrow). MT, middle turbinate.

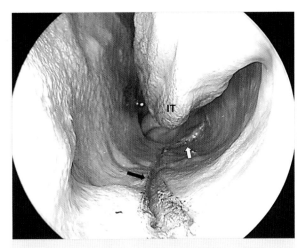

Fig. 12.4 Endoscopic view, 0-degree scope. Inferior (black arrow) and posterior (white arrow) limits of the lateral nasal wall flap. IT, inferior turbinate.

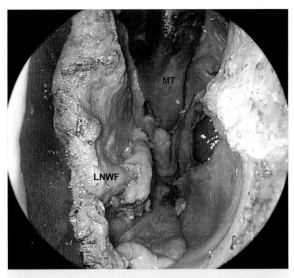

Fig. 12.5 Left nasal fossa, cadaveric dissection demonstrating the lateral nasal wall flap (LNWF) completely harvest and resting over the nasal septum. MT, middle turbinate.

- The inferior incision (▸ Fig. 12.4) goes on the nasal floor from the posterior border of the hard palate to the anterior nasal spine. Then unite the anterosuperior incision with the inferior incision.
- The pedicle's posterior incision joins a sagittally oriented incision that extends over the superior aspect of the inferior turbinate, just inferior to the uncinate process. Posterior to the uncinate process, the incision can migrate superiorly to incorporate the fontanelle of the maxillary sinus. Alternatively, an ipsilateral maxillary antrostomy can be opened to facilitate the previously described incision.
- At the most posterior aspect of this incision, the sphenopalatine foramen and its corresponding arteries will be encountered. In this step it is critical to preserve all the arteries, as the flap will nourish from them.
- The flap is elevated subperiosteally with a Cottle or other periosteal elevator, and the dissection is continued along the medial aspect (bone) of the inferior turbinate.
- The opening of the lacrimal duct is spared by curving the anterior horizontal incision around it or performing an elliptical incision around the opening. Once the incisions around the nasolacrimal duct are completed, the mucosa is elevated medially. It is useful to "greenstick" fracture of the inferior turbinate medially as this facilitates the visualization and elevation of mucoperiosteum from its meatal aspect.
- The remaining mucosa of the lateral aspect of the inferior turbinate and the inferior meatus is elevated, and the residual turbinate bone is removed with rongeurs or through-cutting instruments.
- Once the flap is harvest (▸ Fig. 12.5), the perforation edges are rimmed to obtain fresh margins.

- The flap is sutured with absorbable suture to the surrounding tissue. Usually sutures are placed anterosuperiorly, anteroinferiorly, posterosuperiorly, and posteroinferiorly (▸ Fig. 12.6a, b).
- Silastic sheets are inserted to support the flap and prevent adhesions. The floor and lateral nasal wall are left bare for closure by secondary intention.
- Patients are advised to use saline douches to minimize crust formation.
- Division of the pedicle and suture of the posterior margin of the flap, under general anesthesia, is done 3 months postoperatively.

12.5 Case Example

A 51-year-old man presented with a large septal perforation after a septoplasty 20 years ago. During 15 years he had a septal button, but it was removed because of infection. He presented crusting, dryness, and nasal obstruction. Endoscopic examination revealed a 2.4-cm nasal septal perforation. The CT scan showed an anterior septal defect with limited osteocartilaginous support. Both inferior turbinates were intact and no sign of sinus opacification was shown.

The patient was scheduled for endonasal endoscopic closure of nasal septal perforation with a posteriorly based PLNW flap. Months after surgery, a perfect integration of the anterior portion of the PLNW flap to the nasal septum was observed (Video 12.1). Finally 6 months after the surgery, he was scheduled for endonasal endoscopic surgery to release the posterior attachment of the PLNW flap and close the posterior portion of the septal defect (Video 12.2).

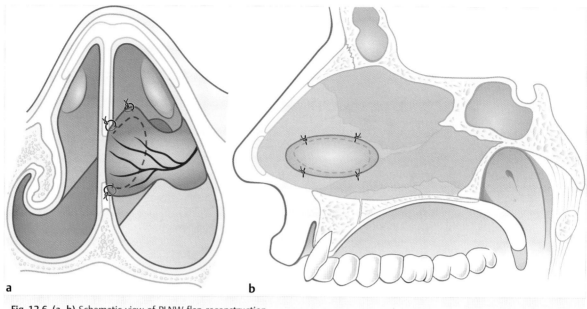

Fig. 12.6 (a, b) Schematic view of PLNW flap reconstruction.

12.6 Discussion

Closing septal perforations is of an extreme complexity so the current medical literature describes countless techniques. Local nasal septal flaps have been the most common surgical treatments for nasal septal perforation up till now.[6,7,8] Kim and Rhee[9] performed a systematic review to evaluate predictive factor for closure success. They observed that the size of perforation was the most significant factor for complete closure. Surgical failure occurred more frequently in patients with large perforation (>2 cm) than those with small to moderate perforation (<2 cm).

The PLNW flap provides a vascularized and healthy wide mucoperiosteal tissue to reconstruct large septal perforation even though there is no osteocartilaginous support. Advantages of the PLNW flap are abundant blood supply and easy rotation. Additionally, the flap consists of respiratory tract mucosa, which allows the repaired septum to achieve normal physiology. The major disadvantage of the PLNW is the requirement for a second procedure to release the pedicle. Another issue is that the flap is bulky and may cause partial nasal obstruction. In addition, the donor surface of the flap must heal by secondary intention producing crusting during the healing process.[6,10] Harvesting of the PLNW flap is not difficult assuming that the surgeon has experience with endonasal endoscopic surgery. However, meticulous attention to its technical harvesting is paramount for a favorable outcome of both harvesting and closure of the septal perforation.

Alobid et al[5] report three patients (55.7 ± 7.5 years; two males and one female) with large septal perforation (34.0 ± 3.0 mm, large diameter) who were reconstructed with the PLNW flap, with complete closure of their defect. All perforations were located in the area of the anterior-mid septum. The donor site was left open for closure by secondary intention during 3 months. All patients complained of variable degrees of nasal obstruction due to crusts mainly on the flap side. Currently there is no other study in the English literature regarding septal perforation reconstruction and PLNW flap, as this technique has recently been described[1] for reconstruction of skull base. Complication and technical hints must be extrapolated of those studies.

12.7 Conclusion

Reconstruction of huge or near total septal defects remains a challenging problem. Using pedicled mucoperiosteal flaps allows for maintaining normal nasal physiology. The current study demonstrates that the PPLNW flaps is a viable alternative to repair symptomatic large defects, as it may cover approximately up to three-quarters of the nasal septum. Familiarity with nasal blood supply and understanding of the potential dimensions of the septal defect allow for more options to correct a difficult problem.

12.8 Complications

See ► Table 12.1.

Table 12.1 Complications and technical solutions

Complications	Technical solution
Bleeding from the PLNA or some inferior turbinate artery while harvesting the flap	Gentle harvest of the flap in a subperiosteal manner to leave the arteries inside the mucoperiosteal flap.
Preservation of the PLNA	Stay 1 cm anteriorly to the posterior insertion of the inferior turbinate.
Infection of the denuded inferior turbinate bone remnant	Remove all denuded bone and/or thorough postoperative care can prevent infection.
Reperforation of the nasal septum	Overcorrect the nasal defect with at flap that is at least 20–30% bigger than the defect as the flap will shrink during the healing process.
Bulky flap that results in nasal obstruction	One can trim the bulky flap with a microdebrider. Use of radiofrequency to shrink the inferior turbinate tissue.
Nasal synechia	Thorough postoperative care removing all the fibrin will prevent synechia.

Abbreviations: AEA, anterior ethmoidal artery; PLNA, posterior lateral nasal artery.

12.9 Tips and Tricks

- Always assess for the osteocartilaginous support surrounding the nasal perforation. If there is no support, one can use the lateral nasal wall flap (LNWF) as it provides enough healthy mucosa to support and cover the perforation.

- Harvest of the flap should always be subperiosteal to avoid damaging the arterial pedicles.
- Stay at least 1 cm anteriorly to the posterior insertion of the inferior turbinate to avoid damaging the PLNA.
- Sharp cut of the nasolacrimal duct reduces the risk of duct synechia.
- Rim the perforation in the final step of the surgery to avoid bleedings during the harvest of the flap.

References

[1] Rivera-Serrano CM, Bassagaisteguy LH, Hadad G, et al. Posterior pedicle lateral nasal wall flap: new reconstructive technique for large defects of the skull base. Am J Rhinol Allergy. 2011; 25(6):e212–e216

[2] Hadad G, Rivera-Serrano CM, Bassagaisteguy LH, et al. Anterior pedicle lateral nasal wall flap: a novel technique for the reconstruction of anterior skull base defects. Laryngoscope. 2011; 121(8):1606–1610

[3] Lee HY, Kim HU, Kim SS, et al. Surgical anatomy of the sphenopalatine artery in lateral nasal wall. Laryngoscope. 2002; 112(10):1813–1818

[4] Wu P, Li Z, Liu C, Ouyang J, Zhong S. The posterior pedicled inferior turbinate-nasoseptal flap: a potential combined flap for skull base reconstruction. Surg Radiol Anat. 2015

[5] Alobid I, Mason E, Solares CA, et al. Pedicled lateral nasal wall flap for the reconstruction of the nasal septum perforation. A radio-anatomical study. Rhinology. 2015; 53(3):235–241

[6] Friedman M, Ibrahim H, Ramakrishnan V. Inferior turbinate flap for repair of nasal septal perforation. Laryngoscope. 2003; 113(8):1425–1428

[7] Teymoortash A, Hoch S, Eivazi B, Werner JA. Experiences with a new surgical technique for closure of large perforations of the nasal septum in 55 patients. Am J Rhinol Allergy. 2011; 25(3):193–197

[8] Islam A, Celik H, Felek SA, Demirci M. Repair of nasal septal perforation with "cross-stealing" technique. Am J Rhinol Allergy. 2009; 23(2):225–228

[9] Kim SW, Rhee CS. Nasal septal perforation repair: predictive factors and systematic review of the literature. Curr Opin Otolaryngol Head Neck Surg. 2012; 20(1):58–65

[10] Yip J, Macdonald KI, Lee J, et al. The inferior turbinate flap in skull base reconstruction. J Otolaryngol Head Neck Surg. 2013; 42:6–11

Chapter 13

Anterior Ethmoidal Artery Septal Flap

13

13 Anterior Ethmoidal Artery Septal Flap

Paolo Castelnuovo, Fabio Ferreli, Pietro Palma

Summary

Nasal septal perforation (NSP) is a defect of the nasal cartilage and/or nasal bone septum with an approximate prevalence of 1% in an adult population, although it has probably been underestimated because many patients remain asymptomatic. There are different surgical treatment options to close the perforation. The authors discuss the anterior ethmoidal artery septal flap. This flap is mainly indicated in symptomatic patients with anterior septal perforation. A unilateral mucosal flap with a large and flexible pedicle should be harvested to bring a suitable blood supply to the flap. The extension to the inferior meatus may create additional mucosal flap, allowing advancement of the flap without tension.

13.1 Surgical Anatomy

Numerous flap designs have been described in the literature to close septal perforations. Advancement or rotation of mucoperichondrial/mucoperiosteal tissue from the nasal septum or nasal floor has been widely utilized.

This study focused on the use of a monolateral mucosal septal flap pedicled on septal branches of the anterior ethmoidal artery (AEA), extended to the nasal floor and the inferior meatus.

Knowledge about the vascularization of the nasal septum is crucial if aiming to preserve its branches during the incision of mucoperichondrium and mucoperiosteum to harvest the septal flap.

Blood supply of the nasal septum occurs through septal branches of the sphenopalatine artery. Here it anastomoses with branches of the palatine and labial arteries and septal branches of the anterior and posterior ethmoidal arteries; they are easily recognizable in the cranial portion of the septum area (▶ Fig. 13.1). An anatomical study on the arterial pattern of the nasal septum, traced by microdissection, demonstrated that AEAs were present in all cases, but the posterior ethmoidal arteries in some cases were absent.[1] These arteries, with the middle septal branch of the sphenopalatine artery and the superior labial branch of the facial artery, mainly contribute to the anastomotic triangle of the anterior septum. Only the posterosuperior area is vascularized by the posterior ethmoidal artery branches.[2] The ethmoidal artery originates from the terminal segment of the ophthalmic artery in the orbit cavity, a collateral branch of the internal carotid artery, and passes between the superior oblique and medial rectus muscle. The AEA then reaches the frontoethmoidal suture through the anterior ethmoidal foramen and enters into the anterior ethmoidal canal along with the anterior ethmoidal nerves. The artery crosses the ethmoid roof diagonally from posterolateral to anteromedial (▶ Fig. 13.2). AEA then divides at the lateral part of the cribriform plate of the ethmoid, giving off two or three branches to the mucosa of the cranial portion of the septum (▶ Fig. 13.3). Finally, they reach the olfactory cleft and supply terminal branches to the olfactory bulb and the meninges.

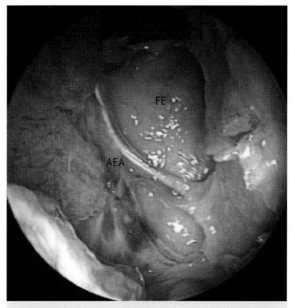

Fig. 13.2 The anterior ethmoidal artery (AEA) identified on the dorsal aspect of the first fovea ethmoidalis (FE) after a complete ethmoidectomy on cadaver specimen (left nasal fossa). The artery crosses the ethmoid sinus diagonally in an anteromedial direction to reach the cribriform plate.

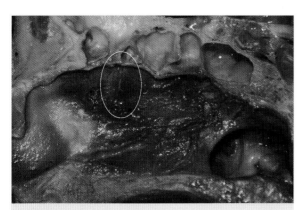

Fig. 13.1 Vascular net of nasal septum in sagittal plane. White circle, septal branch of anterior ethmoidal artery.

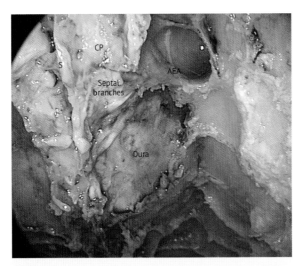

Fig. 13.3 At the level of the cribriform plate (CP), the anterior ethmoidal artery (AEA) gives off two or three branches to the mucosa of the cranial portion of the septum (S).

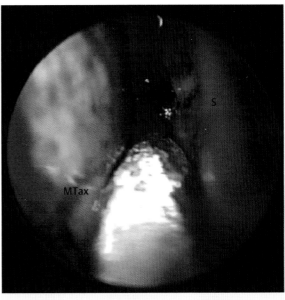

Fig. 13.4 The right nasal fossa. Bleeding can be seen originating from a septal branch of the anterior ethmoidal artery. S, septum; MTax, axilla of middle turbinate.

One must consider that the septal branches of the AEA are at the same level or just posterior to the septal projection of the axilla of the middle turbinate, as confirmed by a recent anatomical analysis, which showed that the average distance was 7.35 mm (range: 5.5–8.7 mm) and never superior to 1 cm.[3]

Bleeding can be seen originating from a septal branch of the AEA, showing a close anatomic relation with the axilla of the middle turbinate (▶ Fig. 13.4). It is extremely important to consider this anatomical relation during harvesting the flap.

13.2 Relevant Analytical Factors

The size and the location of the perforation play a large part in the decision-making process in performing surgery and in choosing the most suitable technique. Symptomatology is essential in determining whether a perforation should be repaired. If the perforation is in the posterior part of the septum and asymptomatic, repair is rarely necessary.

All perforations of our series were located in the anterior part of the septum and the mean size of the septal perforation was 15 mm (range: 10–25 mm).

Based on the anatomical criteria of the nasal septum vascularization, characterized by the constant presence of the septal branches of the AEA, we harvested the monolateral mucosal flap with a large and flexible pedicle to bring a suitable blood supply to the flap. The extension to

the inferior meatus creates a larger mucosal flap, allowing advancement of the flap without tension.[4]

These two aspects, the flap designed without tension and the preservation of the flap's vascular supply, are the main factors contributing to a high rate of closure.

With our technique the normal respiratory mucosa of the nose is used for reconstructing the anatomy and physiology of the nasal septum.

This septal flap is not useful for posterior perforations because the flap cannot be extended to the posterior part of the septum, where the mucoperiosteum is elevated.

Regarding the necessity for bilateral flap provision, monolateral flap coverage was advocated by some authors, as it limits the donor area to one side of the nose, and thus preserves more nasal respiratory mucosa while achieving favorable closure rates.[5,6,7]

Unlike previous studies, a recent case series suggested that NSP could be successfully repaired without using interposing grafts.[8] Even with incorporating grafts, surgical outcomes can vary according to the types of flap utilized for the repair, so the success related to interpositional graft actually is not considered statistically significant.[9]

Furthermore, because no cartilage graft is harvested, it also abolishes donor site morbidity. The choice to use a monolateral flap and avoid interposition of any graft may help reduce operating time.

At the end of the procedure, we recommend the use of Silastic sheets to avoid postoperative scarring.

The endoscopic endonasal approach, in our opinion, is adequate for surgical exposition of anterior septal perforations, flap dissections, and suturing. The use of nasal

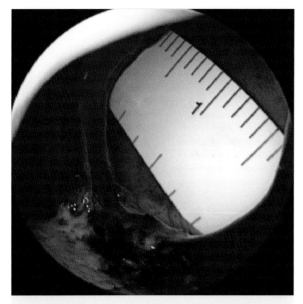

Fig. 13.5 The right nasal fossa. The septal perforation is measured with direct visualization by an endoscope.

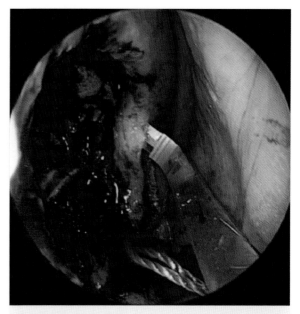

Fig. 13.6 The left nasal fossa. Curettage of all borders of septal perforation achieves a freshening of the edge and promotes a minor amount of bleeding to assist the integration of the flap after suturing.

endoscope allows superior precision in all surgical steps by ensuring excellent access to the operating sites. A critical factor is having a good view of the surgical field and the anesthesiologist's contribution that are essential in achieving an effective hemostasis.

13.3 Surgical Steps

The patient underwent general anesthesia with controlled hypotension.

1. After topical vasoconstriction, a 4-mm, 0-degree rigid endoscope was used to visualize both sides of the nose. The septum and the floor of the nose were injected with Carbocaine (mepivacaine hydrochloride), 1%, and adrenaline, 1:100,000. The perforation was always measured (▶ Fig. 13.5)

2. Curettage of the anterior edge of the septum achieves a "freshening of the edges" effect and promotes a minor amount of bleeding to assist the integration of the flap after suturing (▶ Fig. 13.6). The posterior aspect of the perforation marks the beginning of the superiorly based flap, which contains both mucoperichondrium and mucoperiosteum.

3. Using a Beaver knife (▶ Fig. 13.7a, b), the surgeon fashions the posterior border of the flap vertically along the septum, 1 cm posterior to the septal projection of the axilla of the middle turbinate (▶ Fig. 13.8).

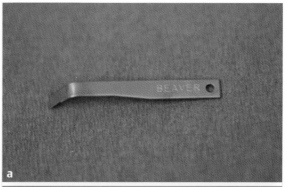

a

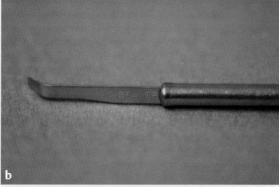

b

Fig. 13.7 Detailed images on Beaver blade (a), with the handpiece (b), which we use to perform the vertical and transverse incision for septal perforation repair with anterior ethmoidal artery septal flap.

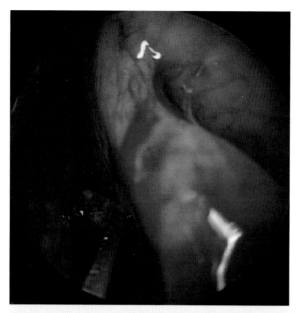

Fig. 13.8 The left nasal fossa. The vertical incision is made 0.5 to 1 cm posterior to the septal projection of the axilla of the middle turbinate.

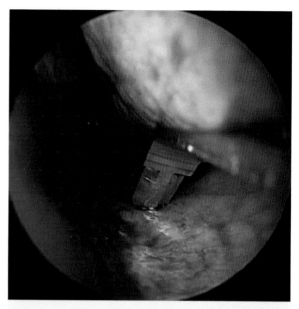

Fig. 13.9 The left nasal fossa. The flap is limited posteriorly by the junction of the hard and soft palate.

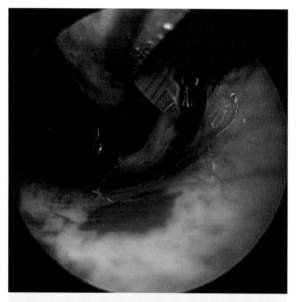

Fig. 13.10 The left nasal fossa. The horizontal incision is extended laterally under the inferior turbinate.

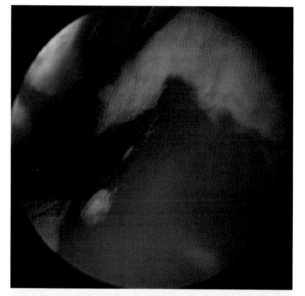

Fig. 13.11 The left nasal fossa. The incision turns parallel to the septum, following the lateral border of the inferior meatus, until it reaches the anterior portion.

4. This incision is continued along the nasal floor, following the posterior border of the hard palate (▸ Fig. 13.9), reaching the lateral wall of the posterior portion of the inferior meatus (▸ Fig. 13.10).
5. Then, the incision turns parallel to the septum, following the lateral border of the inferior meatus, until it reaches the anterior portion (▸ Fig. 13.11).

6. At this point, the incision becomes perpendicular to the septum, reaching the inferior border of the perforation (▸ Fig. 13.12).
7. The extension to the inferior meatus creates a larger mucosal flap, allowing advancement of the flap without tension. Because extensive flap elevation is essential in maximizing the mobility and blood supply of the flap, a superiorly based rotation advancement flap, supplied by the AEA, was developed (▸ Fig. 13.13).

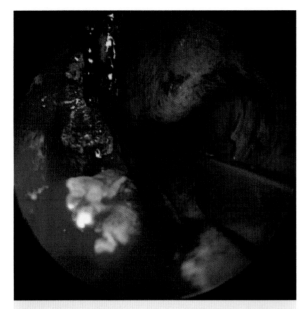

Fig. 13.12 The left nasal fossa. At the end, the incision becomes perpendicular to the septum, reaching the inferior border of the perforation.

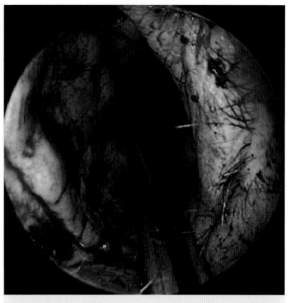

Fig. 13.14 The left nasal fossa. The large mucosal flap is rotated to cover the perforation.

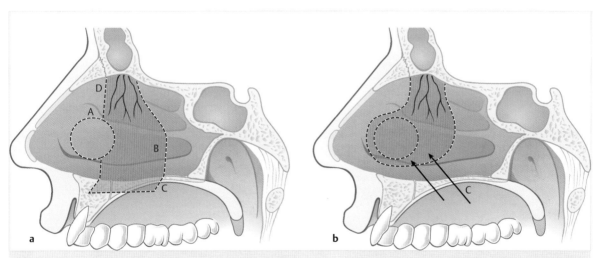

Fig. 13.13 Anterior ethmoidal artery septal flap. The first vertical incision is made at the level of the posterior border of the perforation **(a)**. The second vertical incision is made 1 cm posteriorly to the septal projection of the axilla of the middle turbinate **(b)**. Inferiorly, the incision is extended toward the floor of the nasal cavity, keeping the junction of the hard and soft palate as the posterior border of the incision **(c)**. The septal branches of the anterior ethmoidal artery **(d)** are the main supply to this flap. This design allows the surgeon to fashion a flap of adequate size, pedicled on the septal branches of the anterior ethmoidal artery. Such a flap can be transferred anteriorly, as indicated by the arrows, to cover all the borders of the perforation, with minimal or no tension on the vascular pedicle.

8. The prepared mucosal flap is advanced carefully to cover the perforation, and the posterior portion of the septum and the nasal floor are left uncovered (▶ Fig. 13.14).

9. The surgeon does not make a flap to cover the perforation on the contralateral side (▶ Fig. 13.15).

10. The flap is then sutured to the mucosa at the superior and anterior edge of the perforation, with a reabsorbable suture (polyglactin 910 [Vicryl 5.0; Ethicon Inc.]) (▶ Fig. 13.16).

11. Silastic sheets are inserted bilaterally and left in place for about 3 weeks to avoid postoperative scarring. The nasal cavities are packed with sterile polyvinyl sponges (Merocel), and the packs are removed 2 days after surgery (▶ Fig. 13.17).

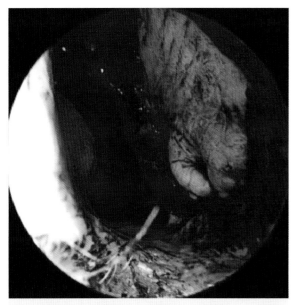

Fig. 13.15 The flap is seen from the right nasal fossa closing the perforation without needing a cartilage graft.

13.4 Complications and Technical Solutions

▶ Table 13.1 discusses points of difficulty and technical solutions.

13.5 Case Examples

13.5.1 Case 1

A 42-year-old woman presented with a long history of mild intermittent epistaxis, crusting and nasal obstruction.

Table 13.1 Points of difficulty and technical solutions

Points of difficulty	Technical solutions
Previous septoplasty	Palpate the septum carefully to anticipate the extent of prior submucosal resection. Take extra caution in elevating the mucosal flaps over absent septal bone or cartilage, or move the incision posterior to avoid dissecting in areas of prior surgery.
Hasner valve in inferior meatus	Make the incision lower than the Hasner valve area. It is important to make the incision by direct endoscopic control of the inferior meatus.
Septal branches of anterior ethmoidal artery preservation	Make the second vertical septal incision 1 cm posterior to the septal projection of the axilla of the MT to preserve these vessels.
Risk of soft palate damaging during the horizontal incision	Palpate the hard and the soft palate to identify the boundary between them.
Posterior deviation with preexisting septal perforation	Make the mucosal incision posterior to the perforation and address the posterior deviation

Abbreviation: MT, middle turbinate.

The patient had several previous nasal septum cauterizations with silver nitrate on local anesthesia and nasal packing for recurrent anterior epistaxis. On physical examination, endoscopic examination revealed an anterior septal perforation, measuring 1.6 cm, with crusts and bleeding areas on the edges, without evidence of suspicious mucosal lesions. Based on the size and the location

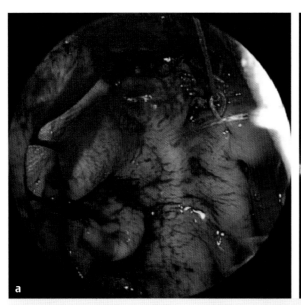
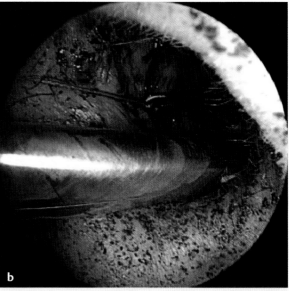

Fig. 13.16 The left nasal fossa. The septal flap is sutured at the superior (a) and anterior (b) edge of the perforation. Two reabsorbable sutures, performed with a curved needle, are sufficient to stabilize the flap.

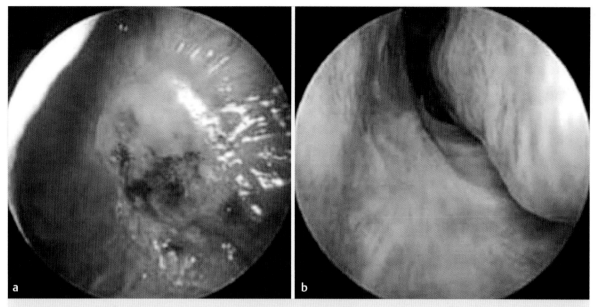

Fig. 13.17 The 6-month postoperative endoscopic views show a complete closure of the perforation (**a**) and the nasal floor is completely covered by nasal mucosa (**b**).

of the septal defect, the patient underwent endoscopic endonasal closure of the NSP by AEA septal flap. The Silastic sheets were left in nasal cavities for 20 days. At 2 years' follow-up, the septal perforations appear closed and the patient reported a complete resolution of symptoms without any more episodes of epistaxis (Video 13.1).

13.5.2 Case 2

A 49-year-old man presented with persistent nasal obstruction, mainly on the left side, and whistling nose. The patient had two previous interventions of septo- plasty. Office endoscopy showed a doubled septal perfo- ration (respectively middle- and small-sized septal defect in the anterior and in the middle portion of the septum) and a left septal spur just posteriorly. The nasal septum was palpated to identify residual cartilage and bone closed to the septal defects. CT scan confirmed the pres- ence of residual cartilage and bone in the posterior por- tion of the septum. Revision of endoscopic septoplasty was performed to correct the septal spur, and also to increase the laxity and the mobility of the septal mucosal layer for the flap. AEA septal flap was harvested to close both septal perforations. One year postoperatively, the septal perforations were completely closed and the defect specific symptoms were significantly reduced (Video 13.2).

13.6 Tips and Tricks

- To avoid a too bulky flap at the level of the cranial part of the nasal septum and in the perforation area, which may partially obstruct the normal airflow, it would be better to harvest a not too wide pedicle. It is enough to perform a pedicle no wider than 1 cm to preserve the artery and, at the same time, to be able to move the flap more easily and with minimum amount of tissue excess.
- It is crucial to obtain a closure of the septal perforation without tension of the pedicle. Over time the scar retraction in anteroposterior direction could compro- mise a correct healing of the mucosa and a subsequent reperforation of the septum at the level of the more anterior aspect of the flap.

References

[1] Chiu T, Dunn JS. An anatomical study of the arteries of the anterior nasal septum. Otolaryngol Head Neck Surg. 2006; 134(1):33–36

[2] Babin E, Moreau S, de Rugy MG, Delmas P, Valdazo A, Bequignon A. Anatomic variations of the arteries of the nasal fossa. Otolaryngol Head Neck Surg. 2003; 128(2):236–239

[3] Gras-Cabrerizo JR, García-Garrigós E, Ademá-Alcover JM, et al. A uni- lateral septal flap based on the anterior ethmoidal artery (Castelnuo- vo's flap): CT cadaver study. Surg Radiol Anat. 2016; 38(6):723–728

[4] Castelnuovo P, Ferreli F, Khodaei I, Palma P. Anterior ethmoidal artery septal flap for the management of septal perforation. Arch Facial Plast Surg. 2011; 13(6):411–414

[5] Newton JR, White PS, Lee MS. Nasal septal perforation repair using open septoplasty and unilateral bipedicled flaps. J Laryngol Otol. 2003; 117(1):52–55

[6] Woolford TJ, Jones NS. Repair of nasal septal perforations using local mucosal flaps and a composite cartilage graft. J Laryngol Otol. 2001; 115(1):22–25

[7] Lee HR, Ahn DB, Park JH, et al. Endoscopic repairment of septal perforation with using a unilateral nasal mucosal flap. Clin Exp Otorhinolaryngol. 2008; 1(3):154–157

[8] Teymoortash A, Werner JA. Repair of nasal septal perforation using a simple unilateral inferior meatal mucosal flap. J Plast Reconstr Aesthet Surg. 2009; 62(10):1261–1264

[9] Kim SW, Rhee CS. Nasal septal perforation repair: predictive factors and systematic review of the literature. Curr Opin Otolaryngol Head Neck Surg. 2012; 20(1):58–65

Chapter 14

Unilateral Mucosal Advancement Flap

14

14 Unilateral Mucosal Advancement Flap

Jung Soo Kim, Sung Jae Heo

Summary

Unilateral advancement flap technique uses one side of mucosal flap from the bottom (inferior-based flap) and the top (superior-based flap) of the perforation of the nasal cavity. The contralateral side, uncovered with the flap, is healed by mucosal regeneration. In general, bilateral advancement flap seems the ideal method for reconstruction of the perforation. Even if mucosal flap of one side fails to close the perforation, contralateral mucosal flap could bring surgical success. However, a unilateral flap has the advantage of shortening of the operative time, and it can be used when the perforation is so large that the flap is hard to cover the perforation simultaneously on both sides. In the case of too large septal perforation, bilateral mucosal flap can cause an iatrogenic, new septal perforation at the site of flap elevation. Therefore, unilateral advancement flap is also a useful method for septal perforation closure.

14.1 Indications

- Almost all of size and shape of septal perforations.
- Patients do not have general inflammatory or vascular diseases.
- The margin of septal perforation is not under the state of infection or inflammation.

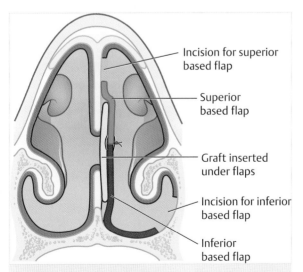

Fig. 14.1 A unilateral mucosal advancement flap technique using inferior- and superior-based flaps on one side of nasal cavity and interposition graft.

14.2 Surgical Steps

14.2.1 General Aspects

Unilateral mucosal advancement flap technique uses two flaps, inferior- and superior-based flap, which are classified by their location in relation to the perforation (▶ Fig. 14.1, ▶ Fig. 14.2). It is easier to develop large flaps from the inferior side of the perforation margin because more usable mucosa and space for handling instruments exist in the inferior nasal cavity. Therefore, the mainstay of the perforation closure is inferior-based flap. To facilitate sufficient mobilization of an inferior flap, incision is needed to be parallel to nasal cavity at the inferior aspect of the inferior turbinate. Dissection of the mucosa at nasal floor allows a maximal mobility of the flap. When more mobility of the inferior flap is required in spite of enough dissection at the inferior nasal cavity, the incision toward the anterior part of the flap, until it reaches the hemitransfixion incision, brings an additional mobility. The blood supply of the flap extended to hemitransfixion

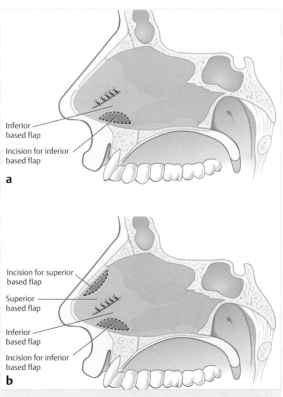

Fig. 14.2 Unilateral mucosal advancement flap using inferior-based flap (a) and both inferior- and superior-based flaps (b).

incision is provided only from the posterior nasal cavity, forming a monopedicled advancement flap. When the flap is getting larger, the risk of a new perforation increases. Especially, a simultaneous development of this flap on both sides has a possibility of a new perforation caused by the exposure of cartilage on the anteroinferior side of the septum on both sides.[1,2]

When the inferior flap cannot sufficiently cover the perforation or achieve a tension-free state at the closure site, a superior-based flap can be used. To harvest a large superior flap, the mucosal dissection is needed to be extended toward the mucoperichondrium at the undersurface of upper lateral cartilage. The mucosal dissection at the superior aspect can be more easily performed by using an open rhinoplasty approach. The simultaneous creation of bilateral superior based flap brings an interruption of the blood supply on the septal cartilage, and it can induce a new septal perforation. Therefore, a precise designing of flap size and location of incision are important factors for a successful closure of septal perforation.

14.2.2 Suturing Techniques

One of challenging part of perforation closure is the suturing of the septal mucosa. When the perforation is located at the anterior part of nasal septum, we can suture the flap using two hands with a direct vision. However, the suturing with two hands is impossible in most of cases of septal perforation, and one hand is used to handle endoscope. One hand suturing and narrow nasal cavity bring surgeons a fear for performing the septal perforation closure. However, our technique described below is simple and easy to learn.

The recommended suture material for the technique is a 5–0 absorbable thread, such as Vicryl, with a cutting needle that can easily penetrate the septal mucosa. The needle pass through both sides of perforated septal mucosa margin under endoscopic viewing and the knot are formed outside the nose, after which the assistant will hold one end of the thread while the operating surgeon holds the other end, at the side of the suture needle, and together they slowly pull on both sides simultaneously. The assistant must watch the monitor to identify that the thread is being properly pulled and then tighten the knot. Subsequent knots are also made outside the nose, but the assistant and the operating surgeon should not pull the tread simultaneously. Instead, the assistant must hold the thread very lightly while the operating surgeon pulls the thread little by little inside the nose to tighten the knot. Suturing must begin in the posterior part and advance anteriorly because, if the anterior part is sutured first, it may disturb the view while suturing the posterior part (▶ Fig. 14.3).

14.2.3 Interposition Graft

An interposition graft is inserted between the two sides of the septal mucosa after mucosal flap suturing, and it increases a success rate of surgery by promoting epithelialization of the sutured mucous membrane. Materials for

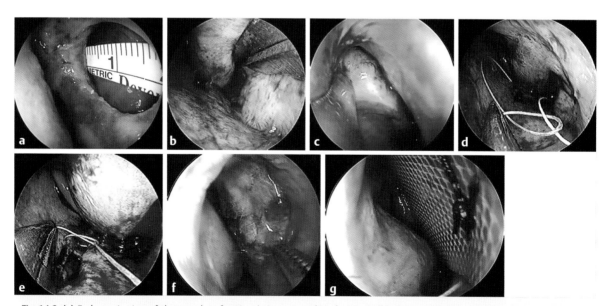

Fig. 14.3 (a) Endoscopic view of the septal perforation (~2 cm size of perforation). (b) The incision for inferior flap needs to be conducted as far as possible to the nasal floor. (c) The incision for superior flap should be performed as close as possible to the nasal roof. (d) The knot is formed outside the nose and loosely it approaches to the perforation site. (e) The assistant tightens the thread with a proper strength and the operating surgeon lightly pulls the thread. (f) Temporalis fascia is inserted at the contralateral side of the unilateral mucosal advancement flap sutured for perforation closure. (g) Placement of Silastic sheet on both sides of nasal septum. It is best to keep the splint for 3 to 4 weeks.

interposition graft consist of pericranium, mastoid periosteum, septal cartilage, septal bone, conchal cartilage, acellular dermal allograft, and so on. The most commonly used graft material is temporalis fascia, and homologous processed fascia can also be used, which does not have much difference from autologous fascia in terms of treatment outcomes. The graft placed between the septal mucosal flap acts as a template during mucosal epithelialization and prevents recurrence of the perforation during healing process. Moreover, a graft fills small gaps that occur during flap suturing. Especially, grafts are useful in cases of unilateral advancement flap because the flap covers one side of the perforation. In general, it is best to make an interposition graft of at least 2 cm larger than or, when possible, twice the size of the perforation.[3]

14.2.4 Insertion of Silastic Sheet and Postoperative Care

When completing suturing and insertion of the graft, Silastic sheets should be placed on both sides of the nasal septum to prevent the mucosal flap from drying, which promotes healing process, and transparent Silastic sheets will permit inspection of the repair site during postoperative follow-up. The Silastic sheet is usually fixed with 5–0 nonabsorbable suture material. The nose should be lightly packed with gauze or Gelfoam, recalling that if the packing is too tight, it may cause necrosis due to interruption of the mucosal blood supply, resulting in surgical failure. Packing needs to be removed on the first or second postoperative day. Because one side of septum is exposed with interposition graft, Silastic sheet needs to be kept for 3 to 4 weeks, and the patients must be instructed to use a humidifier and apply an antibiotic ointment in the nasal cavity three to four times a day.

14.3 Case Example

A 48-year-old man with a large septal perforation visited our hospital. The patient underwent septoplasty 3 years ago at a local clinic. After the surgery, she presented a bothersome whistling sound at the nasal cavity whenever she breathed. She had a repair surgery of septal perforation two times at other institutions, but both surgeries failed and the size of septal perforation increased. Endoscopic examination revealed a 2-cm nasal septal perforation. The computed tomographic (CT) scan showed an

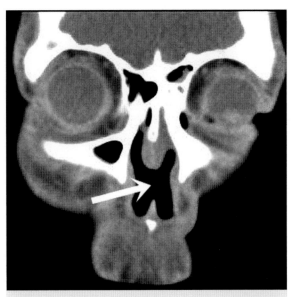

Fig. 14.4 The coronal view of CT scan shows the perforation of anterior nasal septum (white arrow).

anterior septal defect with limited osteocartilaginous support (▶ Fig. 14.4).

The patient was scheduled for endonasal endoscopic closure of nasal septal perforation with unilateral mucosal advancement flap. Months after surgery, a perfect closure of the septal perforation was observed (▶ Fig. 14.5). The symptoms patients complained have disappeared and no recurrence has been found.

14.4 Tips and Tricks

- It is easier to develop large flaps from the inferior side of the perforation margin.
- When more mobility of the inferior flap is required in spite of enough dissection at the inferior nasal cavity, the incision toward the anterior part of the flap, until it reaches the hemitransfixion incision, brings an additional mobility.
- A tension-free state of sutured flap is a key factor for surgical success.
- To harvest a large superior flap, an open rhinoplasty approach is a useful method.
- The suture technique that authors introduced above is easy to learn and perform.

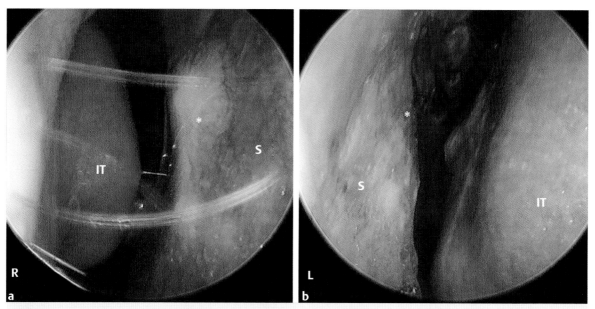

Fig. 14.5 The perforation was completely closed and the mucosa of both sides of nasal septum was well recovered after 3 months from the closure operation. *, the previous site of septal perforation; IT, inferior turbinate; L, left side; R, right side; S, nasal septum.

References

[1] Kim JS, Jang YJ. Septal perforation. In: Jang YJ, ed. Rhinoplasty and Septoplasty. 1st ed. Seoul, South Korea: Kookja Publishing; 2014:100–106

[2] Lee HR, Ahn DB, Park JH, et al. Endoscopic repairment of septal perforation with using a unilateral nasal mucosal flap. Clin Exp Otorhinolaryngol. 2008; 1(3):154–157

[3] Watson D, Barkdull G. Surgical management of the septal perforation. Otolaryngol Clin North Am. 2009; 42(3):483–493

Chapter 15

Bilateral Cross-Over Flap Technique

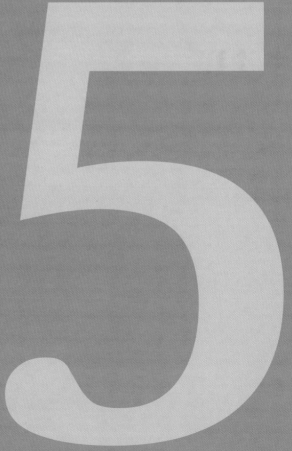

15 Bilateral Cross-Over Flap Technique

Shirley Shizue Nagata Pignatari, Aldo Cassol Stamm, Leonardo Balsalobre

Summary

The correction of a septal perforation can be accomplished by various techniques. Despite the substantial available published literature on the treatment of septal perforations, the optimum technique is not fully established. The choice may depend on the etiology, size, and location, and also the surgeons' preference, although there is a general perception that the size of perforation can be a significant factor for the success of the surgery, as surgical failures tend to occur more frequently in patients with large perforations. Bilateral coverage over the perforation with vascularized mucosal flaps seems also to be a contributor factor for complete closure, when compared to single unilateral flaps techniques.[1,2] The authors describe their technique, the so-called *bilateral cross-over flap technique*.

15.1 Indications

- This surgical technique is conceived to repair medium-sized septal perforations, not larger than 2 cm in diameter.
- This technique can be only accomplished if remaining cartilage covered with mucosa remains above the perforation.

15.2 Preoperative Considerations

- Good visualization (0-degree endoscope) and use of very delicate surgical instruments ensure an easier, faster, and safer procedure. Adequate and delicate instruments are essential to shorten the surgical procedure. In some cases, otologic micro-instruments may be used.
- Every initial step should be directed to prevent unnecessary mucosal trauma and bleeding keeping the edges of the perforation untouched. They will serve as pedicles for the flaps.
- To facilitate tailoring and displacing the septal mucosa flaps, infiltration elevation can be accomplished initially by using a saline solution.

15.3 Instrumentation

- 0-degree scope
- Scalpel
- Suction elevator

15.4 Surgical Steps

The entire surgical procedure can be accomplished with a 0-degree endoscope. Choose the side with more space and more operating exposure. Keep the borders of the perforation untouched.

15.4.1 Step 1. Creation of Flaps

Superior Flap

After proper infiltration, begin by making a racket- or square-shaped incision (right side) beginning at the middle of the perforation anteriorly, extending up beneath the mucoperichondrium of the remaining cartilage superiorly, and making sure the size of the racket or the square delimited by the incision is enough to cover the perforation, and finish the incision at the middle posterior part of the perforation (▶ Fig. 15.1a, b).

Elevate the mucoperichondrial flap carefully without injuring the mucosa that covers the superior half border of the perforation. This flap will cross over the perforation border to the contralateral nasal cavity (▶ Fig. 15.1c).

Inferior Flap

The same shaped incision is made in the contralateral side, beginning at the middle of the perforation anteriorly (just at the same level where the superior flap incision level was made) extending the incision through the floor of the nasal cavity until the inferior meatus, making a racket- or square-shaped flap following the free margin of the inferior turbinate, turning the scalpel back to the septum, and finishing the incision at the middle of the perforation posteriorly (▶ Fig. 15.1d, e). Again, elevate carefully the mucoperichondrial flap without injuring the half inferior mucosal border of the perforation. This flap will pass through the perforation to the contralateral side (▶ Fig. 15.1f).

15.4.2 Step 2. Positioning of Flaps

Very carefully, elevate the mucosa of the edges of the perforation along with the flaps and translocate them; both the superior and inferior flaps go through the perforation to the contralateral sides, and their raw face will face each other to cover the perforation (▶ Fig. 15.2a–c).

The flaps can be kept in position with a loose catgut suture embracing both flaps to the superior cartilage, or just by adding fibrin glue around the flaps bilaterally. Flaps also could be kept in place with a silicone splint, left

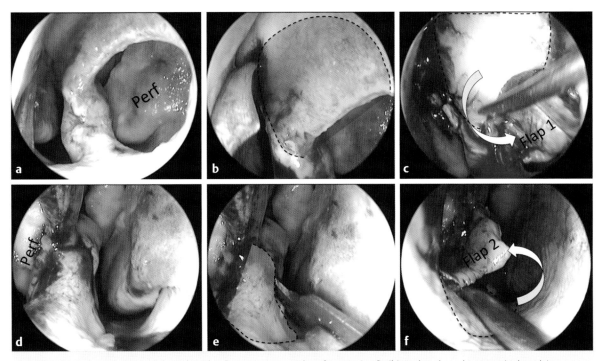

Fig. 15.1 (a) Endoscopic view of the right side of an anterior septal perforation (*perf*). (b) Racket-shaped incision (right side) delimitating the superior flap, making sure that the size of the racket is large enough to cover the perforation area. (c) The superior mucoperichondrial flap (*flap 1*) is displaced without injuring the mucosa that covers the superior half border of the perforation. This flap crosses over the perforation border to the contralateral nasal cavity. (d, e) The same procedure is performed to create the inferior flap: The incision in the *contralateral side* begins at the same level of the perforation border (*perf*), where the superior flap incision level was made, but extending the incision through the floor of the nasal cavity till the inferior meatus, following the free margin of the inferior turbinate, and turning the scalpel back to finish the racket shaped flap. (f) This flap (*flap 2*) goes through the perforation to the contralateral side.

for 4 to 5 days. Two months after surgery, flaps take the final aspect of the septal mucosa (▶ Fig. 15.3a, b).

The authors have successfully operated 11 patients who have presented with iatrogenic septal perforations. One case of failure was observed in one patient with a large septal perforation of unknown etiology.

15.5 Case Example

A 32-year-old woman was referred with complaints of whistling in the nose during breathing. She had undergone a septoplasty and inferior turbinectomy 3 years before. She explained that after the surgery, nasal obstruction improved, but a whistle appeared during inspiration. It had been getting more conspicuous, especially in quiet settings.

Anterior rhinoscopy revealed an anterior septal perforation approximately 1.5 cm in length. Palpation demonstrated septal cartilage around the perforation, especially in the superior edge.

Closure of the septal perforation using a bilateral cross-over flap technique was proposed. The surgical steps are illustrated in Video 15.1.

15.6 Tips and Tricks

- Palpate the edges of the perforation to check for the presence of remaining septal cartilage.
- Infiltrate the submucoperichondrial region before harvesting the flaps.
- Keep the perforation edges untouched.
- Attempt to harvest flaps larger than the size of the septal defect.
- Avoid tension on the suture securing the flaps in place.
- If the first surgical attempt fails, one can always try a second surgery, changing the position of where the flaps were harvested initially in both sides. If a superior right-side flat is used in the first surgery, an inferior right-side flat should be used for the second attempt.

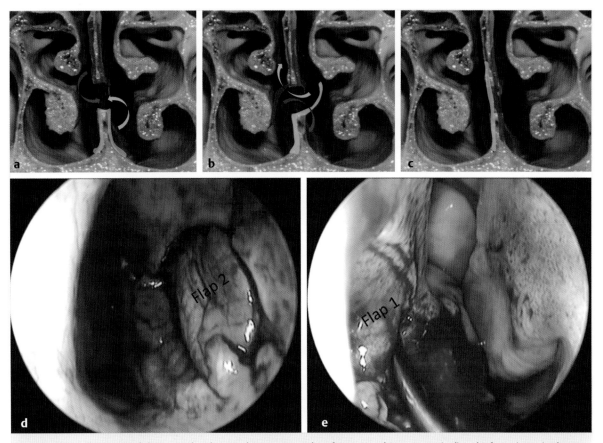

Fig. 15.2 (a–c) Illustration of the surgical technique showing a septal perforation, and its superior (red) and inferior (green) edges covered by mucoperichondrium. The sequence shows how the superior and inferior flaps are displaced, crossing over the perforation borders to have their row side facing each other, covering the perforation area. (d, e) endoscopic view of the *flap 1* (superior) and *flap 2* (inferior), positioned at the end of the procedure.

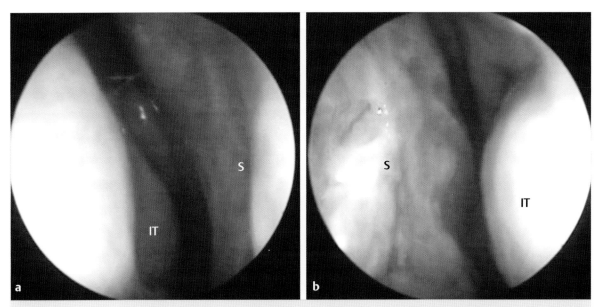

Fig. 15.3 (a, b) Endoscopic view of a 2-month post operation of a septal perforation repair. IT, inferior turbinate; S, nasal septum.

References

[1] Kim SW, Rhee CS. Nasal septal perforation repair: predictive factors and systematic review of the literature. Curr Opin Otolaryngol Head Neck Surg. 2012; 20(1):58–65

[2] Pignatari S, Nogueira JF, Stamm AC. Endoscopic "crossover flap" technique for nasal septal perforations. Otolaryngol Head Neck Surg. 2010; 142(1):132–134.e1

Chapter 16

Bilateral Septal Mucosal Flaps in Septal Perforations

16

16 Bilateral Septal Mucosal Flaps in Septal Perforations

José J. Letort

Summary

Septal perforations repair is a very challenging and sometimes frustrating surgery for the nose surgeon; we describe a technique based on an extended lateral dissection of the mucosa. For this, we can use either the external approach or the endonasal endoscopic approach. The lateral dissection of the flaps extends superiorly under the nasal bones and lateral superior cartilages and inferiorly under the inferior turbinate. For flaps closure, a transfixing suture is preferred to avoid tension and tearing of the flaps.

16.1 Introduction

As a rhinoplasty surgeon, I frequently have to deal with septal perforations in two different situations. First, there are patients with symptomatic perforations due to previous surgery or other previous causes, and second, there are patients in whom the perforation occurs during surgery when the mucosa is bilaterally damaged, which subsequently needs mucosal fixation. It occurs especially in revision surgery.

There are many options to treat nasoseptal perforations, from prosthetics[1] to a number of different types of flaps with or without interposition of tissue. The literature shows the results often contradictory and rarely statistically significant.[2,3]

To repair these perforations, I use a modified technique for hump removal with mucosal preservation. This can be done with an external or endoscopic approach. Both of these techniques need a good dissection of the mucosa and to suture without tension of the flaps.

For this technique, it is very important to know the anatomy of the septum. Review Chapter 3 to get greater insights about blood supply of the nose and nasal septum. Bilateral septal mucosal flaps are dissected in a submucopericodrial-mucopieriosteal plane from anterior to posterior and from superior to inferior, thus preserving the vascular supply of the posterior and superior portion of the septum.

The septal artery network comes from the septal artery that runs over the rim of the posterior choana after the division of the sphenopalatine artery at the level of the sphenopalatine foramen. These arteries run from posterior to anterior so they allow for a good dissection of the bilateral flaps (▶ Fig. 16.1a, b).

The system of the internal carotid artery with one of its branches, the ophthalmic artery, divides into the anterior and posterior ethmoidal arteries, which also play a role in the vascularization of this flap.

16.2 Indications

The advancement of local flaps alone or combined with interposition of grafts techniques is suitable for small to moderate symptomatic septal perforations with good superior and inferior margins.[4]

The main symptoms of nasal septal perforation that we find are crusting, epistaxis, and nasal obstruction, as in the literature. In our patients, these symptoms are worse due to the altitude (2,800 m) and lack of humidity.

Some patients may feel some relief with conservative treatment such as humidification, moisturizing ointments,

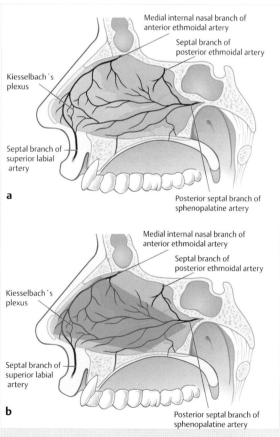

Fig. 16.1 (a) Vascular supply of the septum comes from the sphenopalatine artery and ethmoidal arteries. (b) Drawing of the extension of the dissection (in green) preserving blood supply from sphenopalatine artery ethmoidal arteries.

and nasal saline irrigations; however, these measures have a limited and temporary effect.[5]

Patients with active cocaine abuse, topical nasal vasoconstriction spray overuse (oxymetazoline), systemic disease (granulomatosis with polyangiitis), those who play contact sports, and those who have other similar conditions that impair a good vascular supply are not good candidates for this technique.

16.3 Surgical Technique

The bilateral mucosa flaps technique is based on the septal mucoperichondrial flap, which is insufficient for most of the nasoseptal perforations, and needs to be completed with lateral extension mucoperiosteal flaps in the floor and under the nasal bones. The use of endoscopes is mandatory for the dissection.

Lee et al[6] describe a similar endoscopic technique, but they dissect just one side and use temporalis fascia between the flaps.

16.3.1 Instrumentation

The instrumentation used for this technique is the same as for rhinoplasty when the open approach is used. If we choose the endoscopic approach, a 0-degree endoscope is the standard for mucosal dissection. A 30- or 45-degree endoscope is useful for the lateral extension of the dissection under the nasal bones and in the floor of the nose under the inferior turbinate. For the mucosa edges, a polyglactin (Vicryl) 5–0 is used for suturing.

16.3.2 Technique

Step 1

Local and General Anesthesia

All the patients are operated on under general anesthesia to obtain complete amnesia, analgesia, and sedation. The local anesthesia protocol that we use is as follows:
- Lidocaine 2% in combination with epinephrine 1:200,000
- Oxymetazoline 0.050% embedded in two neurosurgeon pledges

A 27-gauge needle with a 5-cc syringe is used to infiltrate the local anesthetic in the subperichondrial-subperiosteal plane where there is cartilage or bone, and between both mucosa where there is no cartilage or bone. This usually happens around the perforation, especially in the case of postseptoplasty patients. In these patients in whom the loss of cartilage and bone is bigger than the perforation, it is very useful to put the local anesthetic in the right plane to help us with the dissection.

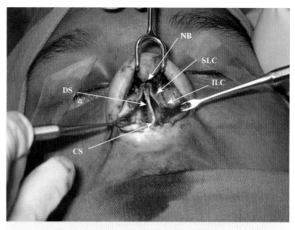

Fig. 16.2 External approach: The exposure of the nasal bones (NB), superior lateral cartilages (SLC), inferior lateral cartilages (ILC), dorsal septum (DS), and caudal septum (CS) makes this approach a good alternative to repair a septal perforation.

We begin the infiltration in the posterior part of the nasal septum and then we continue with small amounts of local anesthetic anteriorly. This helps us to avoid bleeding in the area of injection.

Finally, we inject the floor of both cavities, under the nasal bones and superior lateral cartilages. Cottonoids are placed in each nasal cavity. At this time, the vibrissae are cut with a number 15 blade for maximum visualization during surgery.

Step 2

Approach

External approach: the same technique for open rhinoplasty could be used. Transcolumellar incision is performed, followed by marginal incisions with exposition of the nasal tip cartilages and the dorsum.

A dissection from the anterior septal border to the caudal border is then performed (▶ Fig. 16.2), at this time we have to cut the septum-lateral junction to have a good septal exposure.

In case of the endoscopic approach, we begin with the hemitransfixion incision until we find the submucoperichondrial plane.

Step 3

Dissection

This is the most important surgical step. After finding the submucoperichondrial-mucoperiosteal plane, we begin the dissection of the superior tunnel with the 0-degree endoscope and the Cottle elevator. As soon as we are in the right plane, the dissection is continued with the suction elevator.

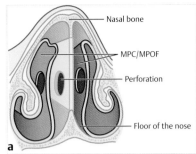
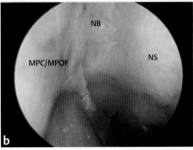
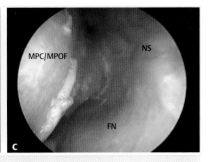

Fig. 16.3 (a) Scheme of the flap dissection (b) and (c) cadaver dissection carried out from the nasal bones (NB) to the floor of the nose (FN). Mucoperichondrial-mucoperiosteal flap (MPC-MPOF) and nasal septum (NS).

The dissection is continued under the nasal dorsum and superior lateral cartilages. For a better visualization, the 0-degree endoscope is switched for the 30- or 45-degree telescope.

The lateral extended superior tunnel is created.

After the superior tunnel is complete, it is easy to continue with the inferior tunnel. For this purpose, the Cottle maxilla-premaxilla approach is used to dissect from the soft tissue lateral to the filtrum until we reach the pyriforme aperture and the floor of the nasal fossa. This step can be done using a headlight instead of scope.[7]

At this time under endoscopic visualization, a 90-degree curved elevator is used to begin the dissection of the floor, and then a suction elevator is used to elevate the mucosa and extend the dissection laterally in the subperiosteal plane in the inferior meatus and under the inferior turbinate.

Finally, endoscopically with the 0-degree endoscope and with the sickle knife, we complete the dissection around the perforation, trying to preserve the mucosa (▶ Fig. 16.3). This step ends when the unified fossa lateral extension is obtained (▶ Fig. 16.4). If there is any septal deviation, we start the dissection in the concave side that is easier to dissect. The same technique is used in the contralateral side.

Step 4

Repairing

For this step, if there is any septal deviation, with the 0-degree endoscope and with the Takahashi through-cut nasal forceps the bone or cartilage deformation is resected.

This correction gives us some extra mucosa to repair the perforation. If the size of the perforation allows us closing without tension, a first attempt to suture the flap in place is done.

The interposition of any type of tissue has been subject of discussion—getting better results with this technique than suturing the mucosa alone in some papers.[8,9] However, other authors find that there is no difference.[4,10,11] Usually we do not use any tissue interposition.

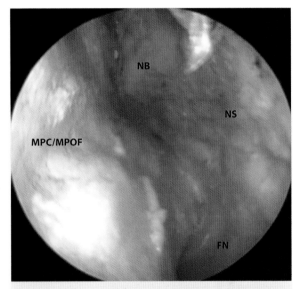

Fig. 16.4 Cadaver dissection of the lateral extended unified fossa, nasal bones (NB), nasal septum (NS), floor of the nose (FN), and mucoperichondrial-mucoperiosteal flap (MPC/MPOF).

If the size of the perforation is too big to close or there is too much tension in the flaps, and if the flap under tension is the inferior, we can make some through-and-through cuts in the floor of the mucosa over the bone.

If the tension comes from the superior part of the flap, the cut should be done under the nasal bones and lateral superior cartilages. The cut must be done with caution, under endoscopic control, and the surgeon has to be sure that there is bone or cartilage behind these cuts.

In some cases, it is necessary to make an incision in the inferior part of the flap from the most anterior part in a posterior direction until there is no excessive tension in the flap.

These cuts can be done with number 11 blade.

Step 5

Suture Technique

Two techniques are possible for suturing the flaps:
1. *Edge to edge suture*: The edges are sutured in each nasal cavity separately using a 5–0 Vicryl. If there is enough mucosa and no tension, it is possible to do this type of technique, but unfortunately this is not the case in most of the patients.
2. *Transfixing suture*: With the same suture, the flap edges are approached in a transfixing way, from one nasal cavity to the contralateral. The advantages of this technique include the following:
   - Less tension in the flaps
   - Less risk of mucosal tear
   - No dead space between the flaps

When necessary, it is possible to combine these two techniques (▶ Fig. 16.5a, b).

The hemitransfixing incision is closed in the case of endonasal-endoscopic approach with 5–0 fast-absorbing interrupted sutures. In the open approach, the marginal incision is closed with 5–0 fast-absorbing interrupted sutures and the transcolumellar incision is sutured with 6–0 nylon.

The exposed bone is left uncovered. The transcolumellar suture is removed at day 7.

Step 6

Packing

If there is some bleeding or if it is necessary to keep the mucosa in place, we use some lubricated packing during 24 to 48 hours. Plastic or Silastic sheeting of the reconstruction is needed to diminish the swelling and help with the mucosa healing. After 2 weeks, the sheeting is carefully removed.

Postoperative Care

The patient keeps his/her nose moist with nasal douches with saline solution and applies antibiotic ointment on both sides of the reconstruction until the healing process is complete.

Antibiotic prophylaxis is done with first-generation cephalosporin (cefadroxil 1 g orally twice a day) before and 7 days after surgery. Alternative antibiotics are used in cases involving penicillin-sensitive patients.

16.4 Complications

The most common complication is septum reperforation. Other less common potential complications include hyposmia, infection, hematoma, vestibular stenosis, and epiphora.[12]

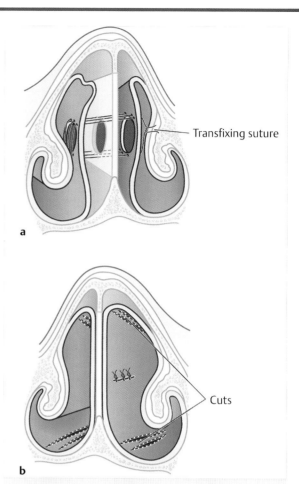

Fig. 16.5 Repairing with transfixing suture from one side to the other of the nasal cavity. (a) Closure of the perforation. (b) Through-and-through cuts in the mucoperichondrial-mucoperiosteal flaps in the floor and under the nasal bones of the nasal fossa. Transfixing suture (TS).

The causes of reperforation include the following:
- Excessive tension in the flaps
- Suture dehiscence
- Infection
- Excessive pressure in the stenting
- Improper candidate for surgery
- Insufficient blood supply

16.5 Case Example

This is the case of a 59-year-old woman, who came to my office complaining of epistaxis, nasal crusting, and post-nasal drip. She had had a septoplasty performed several years before. Apparently, all the symptoms appeared after surgery. Local treatment did not help, so she wanted her septal perforation to be repaired.

The perforation has around 1 cm of diameter with crusting and bleeding. Another smaller perforation was

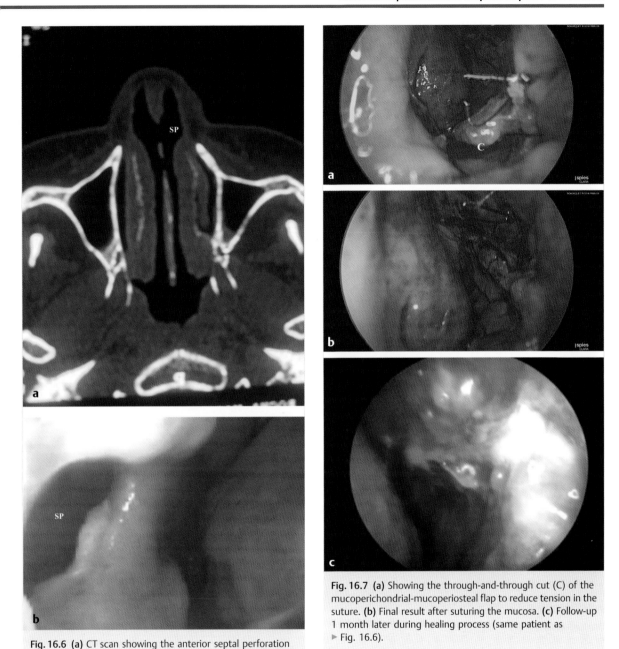

Fig. 16.6 (a) CT scan showing the anterior septal perforation (SP) and the small posterior perforation. (b) Endoscopic vision of the septal perforation.

Fig. 16.7 (a) Showing the through-and-through cut (C) of the mucoperichondrial-mucoperiosteal flap to reduce tension in the suture. (b) Final result after suturing the mucosa. (c) Follow-up 1 month later during healing process (same patient as ▶ Fig. 16.6).

also found behind the first (▶ Fig. 16.6a, b). The suture was done with many transfixing sutures without tension (▶ Fig. 16.7a, b).

16.6 Tips and Tricks

- The bilateral mucosal flaps are a good option for the repair of medium-sized septal perforations.

- The use of endoscope in this technique for the lateral extended mucosal flaps dissection is the key for the success.
- To release, if there is too much tension in the flaps, through-and-through cuts are used in the floor of the mucosa over the bone.
- The key to avoid mucosal tear during the repairing step is the use of transfixing, without tension suture.

References

[1] Taylor RJ, Sherris DA. Prosthetics for nasal perforations: a systematic review and meta-analysis. Otolaryngol Head Neck Surg. 2015; 152 (5):803–810

[2] Goh AY, Hussain SS. Different surgical treatments for nasal septal perforation and their outcomes. J Laryngol Otol. 2007; 121(5): 419–426

[3] André RF, Lohuis PJ, Vuyk HD. Nasal septum perforation repair using differently designed, bilateral intranasal flaps, with nonopposing suture lines. J Plast Reconstr Aesthet Surg. 2006; 59(8):829–834

[4] Kim SW, Rhee CS. Nasal septal perforation repair: predictive factors and systematic review of the literature. Curr Opin Otolaryngol Head Neck Surg. 2012; 20(1):58–65

[5] Lindemann J, Leiacker R, Stehmer V, Rettinger G, Keck T. Intranasal temperature and humidity profile in patients with nasal septal perforation before and after surgical closure. Clin Otolaryngol Allied Sci. 2001; 26(5):433–437

[6] Lee HR, Ahn DB, Park JH, et al. Endoscopic repairment of septal perforation with using a unilateral nasal mucosal flap. Clin Exp Otorhinolaryngol. 2008; 1(3):154–157

[7] Cottle MH, Loring RM, Fischer GG, Gaynon IE. The maxilla-premaxilla approach to extensive nasal septum surgery. AMA Arch Otolaryngol. 1958; 68(3):301–313

[8] Pedroza F, Patrocinio LG, Arevalo O. A review of 25-year experience of nasal septal perforation repair. Arch Facial Plast Surg. 2007; 9(1):12–18

[9] Kridel RW, Foda H, Lunde KC. Septal perforation repair with acellular human dermal allograft. Arch Otolaryngol Head Neck Surg. 1998; 124(1):73–78

[10] Newton JR, White PS, Lee MS. Nasal septal perforation repair using open septoplasty and unilateral bipedicled flaps. J Laryngol Otol. 2003; 117(1):52–55

[11] Dosen LK, Haye R. Surgical closure of nasal septal perforation. Early and long term observations. Rhinology. 2011; 49(4):486–491

[12] Teichgraeber JF, Russo RC. The management of septal perforations. Plast Reconstr Surg. 1993; 91(2):229–235

Chapter 17

Unilateral Nasal Floor and Inferior Meatus Flap

17 Unilateral Nasal Floor and Inferior Meatus Flap

Meritxell Valls Mateus, Cristobal Langdon, Isam Alobid

Summary

The unilateral nasal floor and inferior meatus flap is a simple surgical option for small- to medium-sided nasal septal perforations (NSPs) situated in the anterior and medial part of the septum. Through three incisions, the mucosa of the nasal floor and inferior meatus is freed and rotated medially to fully cover the perforation. This flap has a series of advantages: It utilizes local mucosa, can be used in patients with poor cartilaginous septal support, there is no need for a second surgical time, and the donor surface of the flap heals by secondary intention.

17.1 Anatomy

The floor of the nose is a horizontal structure placed on a slightly lower level than the anterior nares. It is composed of the premaxilla bone and palatine bone in the anterior and middle third and posteriorly by the soft palate.

The nasal floor is a region that receives blood supply from different arteries. The posterior part is fed by the posterior septal artery, also known as *nasal septal artery*, which divides into two branches before reaching the nasal septum. The inferior branch runs toward the nasal floor and is the main artery of this flap. Laterally, this artery anastomoses with branches of the posterior lateral nasal artery, another main branch of the sphenopalatine artery[1,2] (▶ Fig. 17.1). There is also some vascular contribution in the anterior part of the nasal floor and septum from the superior labial branch of the facial artery, which forms the "little area" or "Kiesselbach's plexus" together with the anterior ethmoidal artery and terminal branches of the posterior septal artery.

We measured the dimensions of the nasal floor and nasal floor flap in four fresh cadavers ($n = 8$). The medium length of the nasal floor is 6.03 cm in our samples. The usable area of the nasal floor (between the piriform aperture and the beginning of the soft palate) defines the maximum length of the flap, which is around 4 cm. The medium width is about 2.2 cm with a square area of 8.8 cm² approximately. The width of the flap is modifiable, depending on the size of the perforation, by locating the lateral incision higher in the inferior turbinate or lower in the inferior part of the inferior meatus.

17.2 Indications

- NSPs are situated in the anterior and medial parts of the septum and in the inferior half so the flap can cover the defect completely.

- Perforations in the previously described location of small or moderate size. The vertical dimensions of the defect should not exceed half the height of the septum at that level, because flaps will be mobilized cranially and caudally to the perforation and perforations larger in their sagittal perspective and smaller in their vertical one would be inoperable.[3]

17.3 Surgical Steps

1. Start measuring the size of the NSP to set the extension of the flap. To improve exposure, it can be useful to outfracture the inferior turbinate (▶ Fig. 17.2a).
2. With the 0-degree endoscope, proceed to infiltrate the anterior septum and the floor of the nose with a solution of bupivacaine (0.25%) containing epinephrine (1:100,000) to achieve correct homeostasis and facilitate the subperiosteal and subperichondrial dissection.

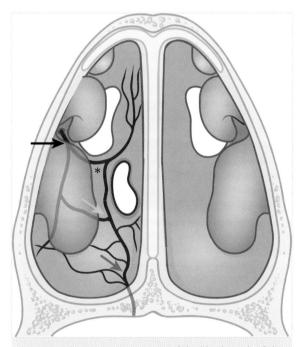

Fig. 17.1 Schematic representation of the blood supply of the nasal floor. The black arrow indicates the sphenopalatine artery giving off the posterior lateral nasal artery and posterior septal artery. The latter divides in two branches before reaching the nasal septum (asterisk). The inferior branch of the posterior septal artery feeds the mucosa of the nasal floor and anastomoses with a branch of the posterior lateral nasal artery (yellow arrow) and more anteriorly with the superior labial branch of the facial artery (blue arrow).

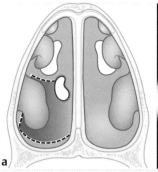
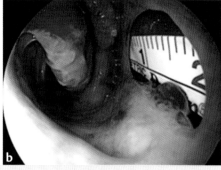
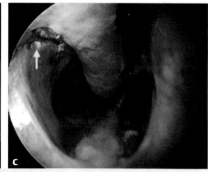

Fig. 17.2 Right nasal cavity. **(a)** The drawing shows the correct placement of the incisions for the nasal floor mucosal flap. **(b)** Location and measurement of the size of the septal perforation. **(c)** Lateral incision along the right inferior meatus (arrow).

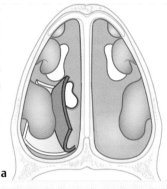
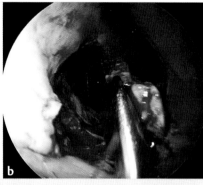
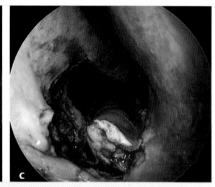

Fig. 17.3 Right nasal cavity. **(a)** Raising of the flap. **(b)** The D scalpel is being used to raise the flap with its cutting edge pressuring against the bone of the nasal floor to avoid mucosal tears. **(c)** The flap along the nasal floor is shown, bended over itself.

3. Incisions (▶ Fig. 17.2b):
   Two parallel incisions are made through the floor of the nose; the first should be located at least 5 mm anterior to the anterior border of the septal perforation, and the second incision at least 5 mm posterior to the posterior border of the perforation.
   a) Anterior incision usually starts in the inferior meatus, at the level of the piriform aperture and it is extended medially along the nasal floor until the premaxilla.
   b) Posterior incision runs parallel to the anterior incision but begins at the junction between the soft and hard palate and, if needed, can be extended laterally to the posterior insertion of the inferior turbinate.
   c) Lateral incision connects the two previous cuts (anterior and posterior) along the inferior meatus. For large perforations, the extended version of this flap including the mucosa of the inferior turbinate can be achieved by placing the lateral incision higher in the lateral wall.[4,5]
      Those incisions can be made with an electric scalpel or a cold instrument, depending on the surgeon's preference. It might be necessary to use sharp scissors to free the flap from the deep fibers at the level of the anterior nasal spine.
4. Avoid mucosal tearing during harvesting of the flap. Verify that the flap is pedunculated at the caudal part

of the septal mucosa to guarantee the blood supply (▶ Fig. 17.3).
5. Rotation and elevation of the flap. Verify the full coverage of the perforation with safety margins (at least 3 mm) to avoid septal reperforation in case of retraction of the flap. (▶ Fig. 17.3, ▶ Fig. 17.4).
6. Rim and refresh the septal perforation edges with a knife until obtaining bleeding mucosal margins (▶ Fig. 17.5).
7. Suturing of the flap. Sutures (synthetic absorbable polyglycolic acid suture; 4–0) should be placed in the superior border of the flap (anteriorly and posteriorly) avoiding tension of the tissue (▶ Fig. 17.6).
8. Verify the total coverage of the septal perforation from the other nasal cavity (▶ Fig. 17.7).
9. Place Silastic sheets in both sides to prevent adhesions and add support while taking care to put them medial to the middle turbinate and without pressuring on the medial attachment of the flap to avoid necrosis.
10. Bilateral nasal packing.

A video showing all the surgical steps has been provided (Video 17.1).

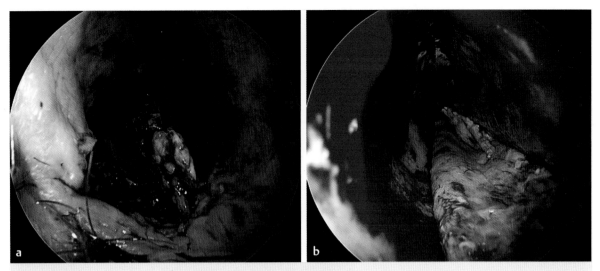

Fig. 17.4 Different stages of raising of the flap in the right nasal cavity.

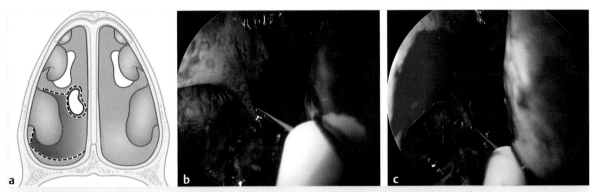

Fig. 17.5 **(a)** Rimming of the septal perforation. Left nasal cavity. **(b, c)** As in tympanic perforations, rimming of the mucosa of the septal perforation, in this case using an ophthalmologic or "Phaco" scalpel to obtain fresh margins and facilitate the integration of the flap tissue.

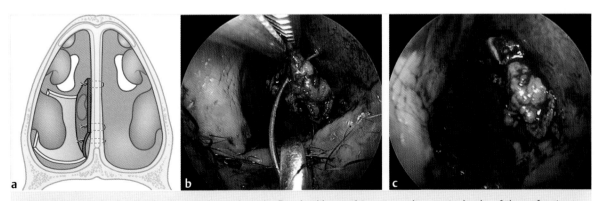

Fig. 17.6 Suturing the flap. **(a)**The drawing depicts how the flap should exceed 3 to 4 mm the superior border of the perforation to avoid reperforation due to tissue retraction during healing. **(a)** Right nasal cavity. Suture of the anterior part of the flap with Vicryl 4–0. **(b)** Appearance of the sutured flap from the same nasal cavity. Notice the anterior and posterior sutures at the superior border of the flap.

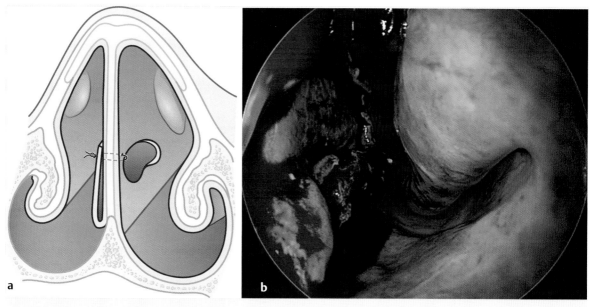

Fig. 17.7 Left nasal cavity. **(a)** Drawing of the final aspect of the flap viewed from the contralateral fossa. **(b)** Intraoperative picture of the appearance of the sutured flap from the contralateral nasal cavity.

17.4 Postoperative Care

Remove nasal packing in 48 hours and take care not to displace the Silastic sheets. After removal of nasal packing, nasal irrigation with saline douches is encouraged three times a day followed by topic vitamin A ointment that helps hydrate and regenerate nasal mucosa after surgery. We recommend following the patient once a week for the first month for thorough aspiration of nasal secretions and removal of crusts. Silastic sheets are removed 2 or 3 weeks postoperatively. The donor surface of the flap heals by secondary intention producing crusts during the healing process.[6,7,8]

17.5 Complications and Technical Solutions

▶ Table 17.1 discusses the points of difficulty and their technical solutions.

17.6 Discussion

Regarding the published English literature, until now there are only two articles from the same author about the repair of NSP using an inferior meatal mucosal flap. In 2009 they described a new surgical technique consisting of obtaining the mucosa from the nasal floor, inferior meatus, and optionally from the inferior turbinate, then mobilizing the flap medially and finally pulling it in a cranial direction through a pouch between the septal cartilage and mucoperichondrial flap.[4] Later, the same authors published a series of 55 patients in which the previously described flap was used to close NSPs achieving a complete closure in 52 patients and a complete symptomatic improvement in all cases.[5]

As mentioned at the beginning of this chapter, the nasal floor mucosal flap has its main indication in perforations under 10 mm with possible application of its extended form using the inferior turbinate for larger perforations. It has the advantage of closing the defect in a single endoscopic surgical step using nasal mucosa.

In Teymoortash's technique, after the clockwise rotation of the flap under the mucoperichondrial septal

Table 17.1 Complications and technical solutions

Complications	Technical solutions
Damaging the soft palate	Meticulously palpate the nasal floor in the posterior part to locate the beginning of the soft palate and place the posterior incision of the flap anterior to this line.
Freeing of the flap in the anterior aspect	Use sharp scissors to release deep fibrous attachments to the anterior nasal spine.
Damaging the superior labial artery	When freeing the flap in the anterior part from the deep fibers, avoid going too close to the nasal spine.
Suturing of the flap	To avoid tension of the flap, harvest enough mucosa to cover the perforation widely.

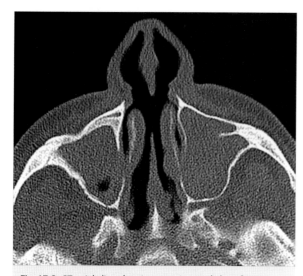

Fig. 17.8 CT axial slice showing anterior-medial perforation about 1.5 cm long and bilateral occupation of maxillary sinus.

flap, nasal mucosa faces the nasal septum, which could lead to formation of mucoceles. In addition, the notable folding of the flap might compromise blood supply. These two aspects are not discussed in his articles and are the reason why we prefer to simply rotate the flap medially (counterclockwise) to cover the perforation.

17.7 Advantages and Limitations

- The unilateral nasal floor and inferior meatus flap allows closure of the nasal septal defect with only one simple procedure in comparison to the inferior turbinate flap that requires a second surgical time, for example.
- The base of the flap along the nasal floor receives blood supply mainly from the nasal septal artery but also from the superior labial artery providing good vascularization for the healing process.
- It can be done unilaterally or bilaterally.

- It can be used in patients with poor cartilaginous septal support (ex: previous septoplasty)
- It is not a bulky flap, allowing correct nasal air flow.
- By using local mucosa, nasal physiology is not disturbed.
- One limitation is in medium to large perforations with history of inferior turbinectomy or medial maxillectomy that would limit the amount of mucosa available for the flap.

17.8 Case Example

A 61-year-old man presented with the history of allergic rhinitis to dust mites in treatment with immunotherapy, aspirin-tolerant asthma, and chronic rhinosinusitis with polyps. Surgical history shows septoplasty and turbinoplasty 15 years ago and polypectomy 3 years ago in another hospital. The patient also explained a nasal trauma with a pencil playing with his son years ago.

The patient complained about anterior and posterior rhinorrhea, crusting, and epistaxis. Nasal endoscopy revealed an anterior septal perforation about 1.5 cm (length) and grade II bilateral polyposis.

The computed tomographic (CT) scan showed pansinusitis and an anterior septal defect with scarce cartilaginous support in the rest of the septum that was also assessed by manual palpation (▶ Fig. 17.8, ▶ Fig. 17.9). Both the inferior turbinates were intact.

The patient was scheduled for endoscopic sinus surgery and closure of NSP with a nasal floor and inferior meatus flap. Surgical steps are illustrated in ▶ Fig. 17.2, ▶ Fig. 17.3, ▶ Fig. 17.4, ▶ Fig. 17.5, ▶ Fig. 17.6, ▶ Fig. 17.7. A short video of the surgery is provided (Video 17.2).

17.9 Tips and Tricks

- To avoid tears when raising the flap, use a surgical instrument (e.g., "D scalpel") with the cutting edge pressuring against the bone of the nasal floor in a uniform way along the length of flap; otherwise, mucosal tears can occur.

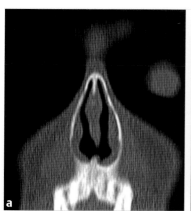
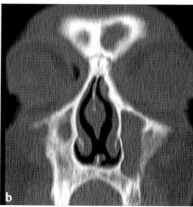

Fig. 17.9 CT coronal slices. **(a)** Anterior slice showing the perforation. **(b)** As in posterior CT slice, the scarce presence of cartilage in nasal septum can be seen.

- Possible options for rimming the perforation are the ophthalmologic "Phaco" scalpel that has a small malleable blade or a conventional number 11 blade.
- Remember that the posterior lateral nasal artery (branch of the sphenopalatine artery) enters the inferior turbinate on the superior aspect of its lateral attachment between 1.0 and 1.5 cm from its posterior tip. Then, this artery enters a bony canal and bifurcates into two branches.[8] One branch remains high and lateral, whereas the other runs in a lower and more medial position, which could be the source of bleeding when performing the posterior incision of the nasal floor mucosal flap.

References

References in bold are recommended readings.

[1] Zhang X, Wang EW, Wei H, et al. **Anatomy of the posterior septal artery with surgical implications on the vascularized pedicled nasoseptal flap. Head Neck. 2015; 37(10):1470–1476**

[2] Lee HY, Kim HU, Kim SS, et al. Surgical anatomy of the sphenopalatine artery in lateral nasal wall. Laryngoscope. 2002; 112(10):1813–1818

[3] Neumann A, Morales-Minovi CA, Schultz-Coulon HJ. [Closure of nasal septum perforations by bridge flaps] [in Spanish]. Acta Otorrinolaringol Esp. 2011; 62(1):31–39

[4] Teymoortash A, Werner JA. **Repair of nasal septal perforation using a simple unilateral inferior meatal mucosal flap. J Plast Reconstr Aesthet Surg. 2009; 62(10):1261–1264**

[5] Teymoortash A, Hoch S, Eivazi B, Werner JA. **Experiences with a new surgical technique for closure of large perforations of the nasal septum in 55 patients. Am J Rhinol Allergy. 2011; 25(3):193–197**

[6] Friedman M, Ibrahim H, Ramakrishnan V. Inferior turbinate flap for repair of nasal septal perforation. Laryngoscope. 2003; 113(8):1425–1428

[7] Yip J, Macdonald KI, Lee J, et al. The inferior turbinate flap in skull base reconstruction. J Otolaryngol Head Neck Surg. 2013; 42:6–11

[8] Alobid I, Mason E, Solares CA, et al. Pedicled lateral nasal wall flap for the reconstruction of the nasal septum perforation. A radio-anatomical study. Rhinology. 2015; 53(3):235–241

Chapter 18

Facial Artery Musculomucosal Flap

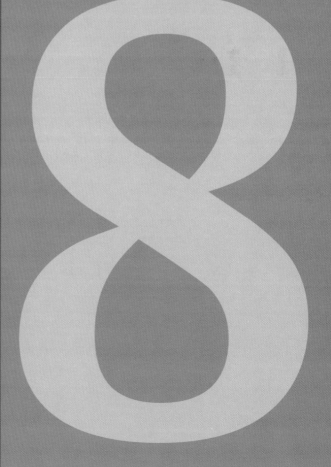

18 Facial Artery Musculomucosal Flap

Tareck Ayad, Philippe Lavigne, Ilyes Berania

Summary

The facial artery musculomucosal (FAMM) flap is a versatile locoregional pedicled flap that has gained popularity in reconstructive surgery. When tunneled into the nasal cavity, it provides plentiful vascularized tissue for larger septal perforation. Although technically challenging, it is associated with low morbidity and leaves no visible external scar.

18.1 Introduction

Over the past decades, regional pedicled flaps have increasingly been used to restore small- to medium-sized defects of the head and neck including nasal septum perforations. While small symptomatic perforations are traditionally closed by local mucosal flap,[1,2] the facial artery musculomucosal (FAMM) flap has become a popularized technique for the repair of large symptomatic septal defects (> 2–3 cm).[3] Other reconstructive options such as open rhinoplasty approaches,[4,5,6,7,8,9,10,11,12] nasal tissue expanders,[13] forearm free flap,[14] and pericranial flaps[15] have also been used for large septal deficits. Initially described in 1992 by Pribaz et al,[16] the FAMM flap is a relatively simple and timesaving procedure that avoids residual external scars of the face.[17]

In this chapter, we describe and review an endonasal surgical approach using a pedicled flap, the superiorly based FAMM flap, as an alternative option for correction of large nasal septal perforation (NSP).

18.2 Indications

- Large septal perforations (≥ 2 cm)
- Septal perforation in patients with poor quality or lack of intranasal tissues such as those with previous radiation therapy in the concerned area, extensive ablative surgeries, or chronic cocaine abuse

18.3 Anatomy

18.3.1 Facial Artery Pedicle

The facial artery follows a cervical course after exiting the external carotid artery. It crosses the submandibular gland and reaches the inferior border of the mandible at the anterior limit of the masseter muscle. The facial artery travels in the cheek lateral to the buccinator muscle and the *levator anguli oris*, while remaining medial to the *risorius*, *zygomaticus major*, and the superficial layer of the *orbicularis oris* muscle.[18,19] The artery has a very tortuous trajectory on its way to the internal canthus to form the angular artery. Through this latter we can expect a retrograde flow from the ophthalmic artery, which originates from the internal carotid artery system.[20]

The facial artery is located approximately 16 mm from the labial commissure. It sends off perforators of the jugal area and branches to give the superior labial artery among others. Several branching variations and terminal endings of the facial artery have previously been described.[21] The classification by Lohn et al includes[22] type I = angular, type II = lateral nasal, type III = alar, type IV = superior labial, type V = inferior labial, and type VI = undetected.

The facial vein usually runs posteriorly and in close proximity to the facial artery at the level of the mandible. It progressively diverges from the artery as it reaches the nose. Doppler flow studies have shown an average distance between the two vessels of 13.6 mm at the oral commissure and 16.3 mm under the alar base.[23] The vein begins at the internal canthus as the angular vein and runs along the nasogenian fold to become the facial vein.

18.3.2 Facial Artery Musculomucosal Flap

The FAMM flap is an intraoral cheek flap and includes the buccal mucosa, submucosa, buccinator muscle, and superficial layer of the *orbicularis oris* muscle (▶ Fig. 18.1). Superiorly based flaps are used for nasal septum perforations to maximize tissue length. Superiorly based FAMM flaps are pedicled on the angular artery and perfusion occurs through a retrograde flow. The facial artery is preserved on the entire length for the flap and kept attached to the buccinator muscle (▶ Fig. 18.2). The facial vein is usually not included in the flap as venous drainage is assured by a submucosal plexus.[24] The pivot point of flap is in the vicinity of the maxillary tuberosity or in the gingivolabial sulcus. The average width of the flap is 2.5 to 3 cm, and the pedicle base should be at least 1.5 cm to ensure adequate venous drainage.[17]

18.4 Surgical Technique

The FAMM flap was first described by Pribaz et al in 1992[16] as a versatile musculomucosal flap harvested intraorally in the area of the jugal mucosa. It can be pedicled either inferiorly on the facial artery or superiorly on the angular artery. For the reconstruction of intranasal defects, a superiorly based pedicled FAMM flap will be harvested.

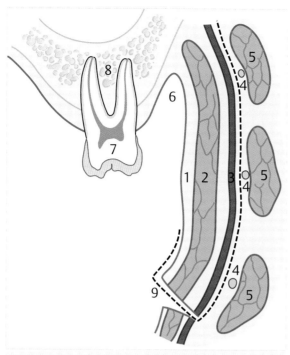

Fig. 18.1 Schematic illustration of the FAMM flap in a coronal cut through the cheek. (1) Mucosa and submucosa; (2) buccinator muscle; (3) facial artery; (4) motor branches of the facial nerve; (5) mimic facial muscles; (6) superior gingivobuccal sulcus; (7) molar; (8) maxilla; (9) incision and plane of dissection of the FAMM flap (interrupted line).

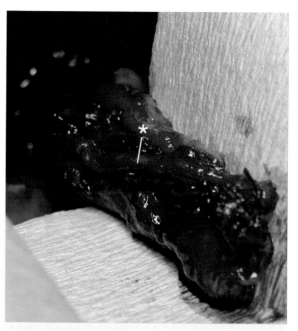

Fig. 18.2 Example of a facial artery preserved on the entire length of the FAMM flap. *, course of the facial artery.

18.4.1 Anesthesia

Antimicrobial prophylaxis directed against oral cavity flora is recommended. After oral intubation, the endotracheal tube is positioned contralateral to the surgical bed. It can be held in place with transjugal or intraoral dental sutures. Neuromuscular-blockage will facilitate exposure of the oral cavity throughout the procedure. We do not recommend local infiltration of the flap outline with an epinephrine solution as it can provoke a spasm of the facial artery that may hinder its dissection.

18.4.2 Drawing the Flap

The buccal mucosa is exposed using two traction sutures in the upper and lower lips and a Weider's tongue retractor (heart-shaped). Alternatively, Senn's retractors or Gillies skink hooks can be used instead of traction sutures. With the anatomical landmarks in mind, an outline of the flap is drawn on the buccal mucosa (▶ Table 18.1). The anterior limit of the flap lays 1 cm posterior to the labial commissure to avoid its distortion after closure of the defect. The posterior limit of the flap lies just anterior to Stensen's duct papillae. A distance of 0.5

to 1 cm is preserved between the posterior margin of the flap and the gingiva to facilitate wound closure (▶ Fig. 18.3). The use of a Doppler to identify the facial artery has been previously described[3] but will hardly ever modify the flap outline, as it relies on fixed anatomical landmarks. Moreover, the facial artery course outline is not reliable anymore after the mucosal incision because the mucosa becomes loose. Superiorly, the flap base is designed to hinge at the junction between the gingivolabial sulcus and first molar.

The distal end of the flap is designed according to the size and shape of the septal perforation. Measurement of the defect or usage of a template is mandatory and will allow an optimal flap outline. As the width of the FAMM flap is limited by the aforementioned landmarks (usually ~3 cm), the size and axis of the defect will decide whether

Table 18.1 Anatomic pearls and their implication

Anatomical landmark	Surgical implication
Lip commissure	Anterior limit (1 cm from the commissure)
Stensen's papillae	Posterior limit
Gingivolabial sulcus	Pivot point
Facial artery	Lateral (superficial) wall of the artery defines the depth of the dissection plane
Y junction between facial and superior labial arteries	Superior labial artery can be identified first and dissected backward to identify the facial artery

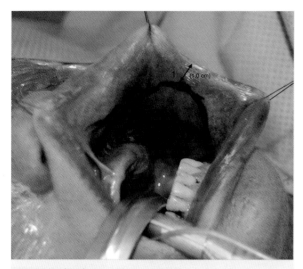

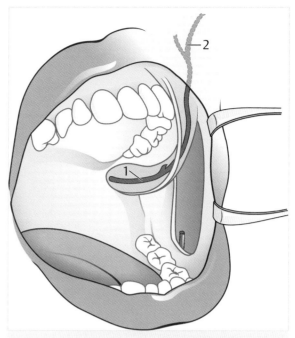

Fig. 18.3 Flap design with anatomical landmarks. (1) A distance of 1 cm is preserved between the anterior portion of the flap and the labial commissure; (2) Stensen's duct papillae is visualized posteriorly to the flap; (3) the distal portion of the flap is pointing toward the gingivolabial sulcus; (4) a minimal width of 1.5 cm is conserved at the base of the flap; (5) a distance of 0.5 to 1 cm is preserved between the posterior margin of the flap and the gingiva to facilitate wound closure.

Fig. 18.4 Superiorly based FAMM flap. The distal portion of the flap is designed to hinge at the junction between the gingivolabial sulcus and the first molar. (1) Facial artery; (2) superior labial artery.

the flap's inset will be horizontal or vertical. For a long craniocaudal perforation, the flap's inset will be horizontal, whereas a tall-vertical perforation will be covered with the flap inserted vertically.

18.4.3 Facial Artery Identification

The facial artery can be identified with two techniques. First, it can be located with careful blunt dissection at the distal end of the flap (▶ Fig. 18.4). Alternatively, the superior labial artery will be identified first with an incision in the area of the labial commissure and then traced back in a retrograde manner to the facial artery. It is only when the facial artery is identified that the superior labial artery is ligated.

18.4.4 Flap Harvest

The mucosal incisions are completed according to the previously drawn outline and extend through the mucosa, submucosa, and buccinator muscle. The flap is harvested in a plane deep to the facial artery. The facial artery must be kept attached to the overlying buccinator muscle over its entire length throughout the dissection (see ▶ Fig. 18.1). The facial artery is dissected in a retrograde manner, from distal to proximal. This warrants meticulous dissection as the artery is tortuous and collateral vessels will need to be clipped. As previously mentioned, the facial vein is not included as venous drainage relies on the submucosal plexus.

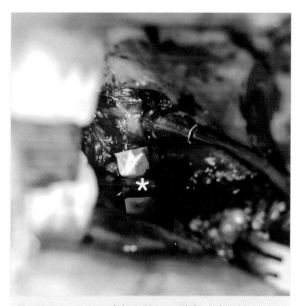

Fig. 18.5 Front view of the oral cavity (left). *, facial artery is identified at the distal portion of the flap (resting on a blue paper).

18.4.5 Distal Flap Preparation

The FAMM flap is fully dissected up to its base, at the junction of the gingivolabial sulcus and first molar (▶ Fig. 18.5). The distal end of the flap now has a mucosal

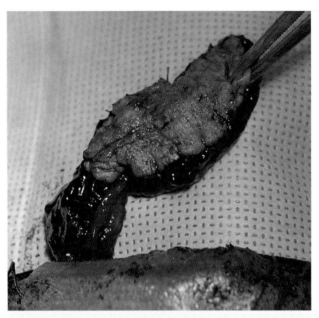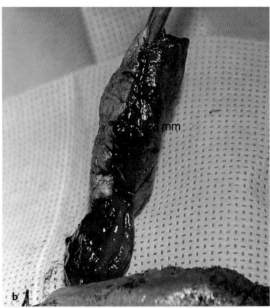

Fig. 18.6 **(a)** A skin graft is sutured circumferentially on the muscular surface of the flap. **(b)** Side view of the flap. A raw muscular surface (2–3 mm) must be preserved at the perimeter of the flap to allow optimal healing against the septal perforation edges.

side and a muscular side (buccinator muscle). The muscular side has to be covered with a full-thickness postauricular or supraclavicular skin graft prior to the flap inset (▶ Fig. 18.6a) The size of the skin graft is based on a template of the septal perforation size and shape. It is attached to the muscular side of the FAMM flap with a running absorbable suture. A raw muscular surface must be preserved at the perimeter of the flap to allow optimal healing against the septal perforation edges (▶ Fig. 18.7b).

18.4.6 Flap Inset

The gingivolabial sulcus is incised by extending the flap's posterior edge and the dissection is deepened up to the inferior border of the pyriform aperture. A subperiosteal tunnel is created to the floor of the nasal cavity with a freer. The flap is tunneled into the nasal cavity though a 2-cm incision on the nasal floor mucosa. The flap is then inset horizontally or vertically as previously described (▶ Fig. 18.7). The posterior edge of the flap is sutured thoroughly to the posterior septal cartilage or bone using an endoscope and absorbable sutures. Small holes can be drilled through the vomer and/or the perpendicular plate, with a right-angle drill to facilitate suture passage for posterior flap attachment. The anterior flap is sutured similarly using a nasal speculum or an endoscope (▶ Fig. 18.8). During the inset, the surgeon needs to be attentive of the facial artery's position in the flap as a misplaced suture could endanger the flap's perfusion (▶ Fig. 18.9).

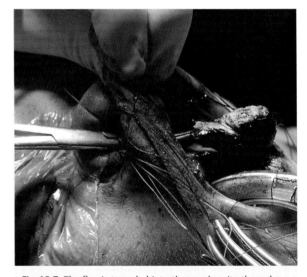

Fig. 18.7 The flap is tunneled into the nasal cavity through a 2-cm incision on the nasal floor mucosa. Handling and positioning of the flap should be done cautiously to avoid torsion of the pedicle.

18.4.7 Closure of Donor Site

Donor site is closed primarily with interrupted mattress sutures using chromic or PDS (polydioxanone) sutures when the flap is less than 3 cm wide.[25] Larger defects can cause labial contracture if closed primarily and can be closed with a skin graft, left to granulate[26] or closed with

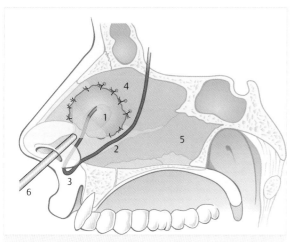

Fig. 18.8 Septal view of the inset FAMM flap. (1) The flap was tunneled into the nasal cavity, positioned into the large septal defect and sutured into place; (2) course of the facial artery; (3) superior gingivolabial sulcus; (4) posterior and inferior sutures were placed through the perpendicular plate via drill holes to secure the flap; (5) vomer bone; (6) anterior flap is sutured similarly using an endoscope.

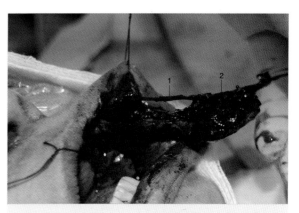

Fig. 18.9 Situation to avoid. (1) Facial artery is separated from the buccinator muscle at the proximal portion of the flap; (2) the distal end of the vessel remains attached to the flap. Tissue may remain viable, but cautious inspection of flap perfusion should be assessed.

buccal fat pad advancement.[27] In the setting of septal perforation repair, this situation is rarely encountered.

The communication between the oral and nasal cavities should be closed primarily to avoid an oronasal fistula. This delicate step requires superficial incision of the mucosa of the flap at its base to allow closure of the communication over raw edges. It is of utmost importance to keep this incision superficial to avoid compromising the submucosal venous plexus and thus avoid venous congestion of the flap. We do not hesitate to delay closure of the communication between nasal and oral cavities for 3 weeks to avoid a possible venous compromise. However, if the septal reconstruction is part of a more complex nose reconstruction involving cartilage or bone grafts, we recommend closing the oronasal communication without delay.

18.4.8 Postoperative Care

The nasal cavity is packed with Surgifoam rather than nasal ribbon gauze or nasal splints that could create an ischemic pressure on the flap or its pedicle. Nasal packing is removed 7 to 10 days postoperatively. We recommend postoperative use of antibiotics for 1 week. If needed, the pedicle can be safely sectioned 3 weeks after the initial surgery.[25]

18.5 Contraindications

The use of the FAMM flap should be discouraged in the presence of buccal mucosa precancerous or cancerous lesions for obvious reasons.[28] Any procedure that could compromise the retrograde arterial blood flow is a contraindication for a superiorly based FAMM flap. Prior facial artery embolization or reconstructive flaps based on the angular artery could interrupt the retrograde blood flow to the flap. The use of a Doppler to assess blood flow is not reliable in these situations as it could reflect inputs from the external carotid artery system or collateral contributions from the contralateral mental, inferior labial, and superior labial arteries.[29] During the dissection, these collateral vessels will be ligatured as the arterial vascularization of the flap depends mostly on the angular artery.

Previous radiation therapy in the surgical field is commonly associated with higher complications rates in reconstructive surgery and should also be considered as a relative contraindication. Retrospective series have shown higher rates of trismus, dehiscence, and necrosis for FAMM flaps harvested in a previously radiated area.[25,26,30]

18.6 Discussion

In their systematic review, Ayad and Xie[25] reported the use of the FAMM flap as a reconstructive flap in 485 head and neck surgery cases. Of these, only 8 (1.8%) were used for septal perforation repair. Other sites of reconstruction studied in this review were the floor of mouth, palate, alveolar ridge, lip, oropharynx, tongue, and buccal mucosa. Taken altogether, the reported complications included partial distal necrosis (12.2%), complete necrosis (2.9%), and "other complications" (12.8%) (dehiscence, venous congestion, hematoma, and infections). There were three reported cases of temporary facial paralysis, all of which resolved within 2 months. Unfortunately, this study did not review the success rates of closure in the cases of NSP specifically, yet the FAMM flap achieved good functional outcomes with defects reconstructed with a superiorly or inferiorly based FAMM flap.

A single peer-reviewed article has been published on the use of the FAMM flap solely in NSP repair.[3] In their work, Heller et al found a 100% success rate (six patients) in closure of the septal defect ranging from 3.1 to 4 cm in greatest dimension. All patients had complete resolution of their discomfort at long-term follow-up (10–30 months) and no complications were reported.

Ferrari et al reported the use of a superiorly based FAMM flap in 12 head and neck defect reconstructions, of which 2 were used for nasal septal defect repair. Overall, authors reported low rates of minor complications (small dehiscence, partial necrosis, congestion) and no major complications. In their septal perforation repair cases, no complications were reported and the defect remained closed at long-term follow-up (11 and 25 months).

Hence, the FAMM flap appears to be a safe procedure for reconstruction of head and neck tissue defects, yet its use in NSP repair remains uncommon. With the rising popularity of this flap[25] in recent years, further studies might confirm its place in the algorithm for NSP repair.

18.7 Case Example

A 44-year-old woman was referred with a diagnosis of symptomatic septal perforation despite an optimal medical treatment. She suffered of nasal crusting, epistaxis, and nasal discomfort. She had used cocaine in the past and explained that the symptoms persisted even though she stopped cocaine usage for the last three years.

Anterior rhinoscopy revealed an anterior septal perforation measuring 2 cm in a cephalocaudal plane and 3 cm anteroposteriorly. The remnant nasal mucosa looked fibrotic.

Closure of the septal perforation using an FAMM flap was proposed considering the size of the perforation and the poor quality of the remaining nasal mucosa. The key steps are illustrated through the Figs. 18.3, 18.4, 18.5, 18.6, 18.7 and 18.8.

18.8 Complications

▶ Table 18.2 discusses the complications and related technical solutions.

18.9 Tips and Tricks

- Design the flap respecting the landmarks described earlier. If the width of the flap needs to be made smaller, do not place the anterior incision more posteriorly as the facial artery is close to the 1 cm mark from the labial commissure. Instead, draw the posterior incision further away (anteriorly) from Stensen's duct.
- Incise the buccal mucosa with a needle tip cautery in "cut" mode to lessen bleeding. We do not recommend

Table 18.2 Complications and technical solutions

Complications	Technical solutions
Facial artery is separated from the buccinator muscle during the dissection.	Careful dissection lateral to the facial artery with care to leave the artery attached to the muscle on the whole flap length.
Facial artery is damaged close to the base of the flap during dissection.	The defective flap can be sutured back to its surgical bed. A contralateral FAMM flap can be used.
Difficult facial artery identification with an initial distal incision.	Identification of the superior labial artery and retrograde dissection up to the facial artery
Posterior suturing of the flap through the vomer bone.	Small holes can be drilled through the bone to allow passage of sutures for the posterior attachment of the flap.
Excessive tension when closing surgical bed.	Cheek fat pad advancement flap sutured to the edges of the primary defect.

Abbreviation: FAMM, facial artery musculomucosal.

infiltration with lidocaine and epinephrine as the facial artery may spasm and become hard to locate.
- Harvest a flap a few millimeters larger than the perforation.
- The shortest way to an anterior septal perforation is through a gingivolabial incision directly toward the floor of the nose. Do not try to use a transmaxillary approach as it will create undue tension on the flap.
- If the first surgical attempt fails, one can always try a second surgery. However, the reason underlying the failure should be identified before a second attempt.

References

References in bold are recommended readings.

[1] Fairbanks DN. Closure of nasal septal perforations. Arch Otolaryngol. 1980; 106(8):509–513

[2] Karlan MS, Ossoff RH, Sisson GA. A compendium of intranasal flaps. Laryngoscope. 1982; 92(7 Pt 1):774–782

[3] **Heller JB, Gabbay JS, Trussler A, Heller MM, Bradley JP. Repair of large nasal septal perforations using facial artery musculomucosal (FAMM) flap. Ann Plast Surg. 2005; 55(5):456–459**

[4] Newton JR, White PS, Lee MS. Nasal septal perforation repair using open septoplasty and unilateral bipedicled flaps. J Laryngol Otol. 2003; 117(1):52–55

[5] van Kempen MJ, Jorissen M. External rhinoplasty approach for septal perforation. Acta Otorhinolaryngol Belg. 1997; 51(2):79–83

[6] Kridel RW, Appling WD, Wright WK. Septal perforation closure utilizing the external septorhinoplasty approach. Arch Otolaryngol Head Neck Surg. 1986; 112(2):168–172

[7] Romo T, III, Foster CA, Korovin GS, Sachs ME. Repair of nasal septal perforation utilizing the midface degloving technique. Arch Otolaryngol Head Neck Surg. 1988; 114(7):739–742

[8] Arnstein DP, Berke GS. Surgical considerations in the open rhinoplasty approach to closure of septal perforations. Arch Otolaryngol Head Neck Surg. 1989; 115(4):435–438

[9] Teichgraeber JF, Russo RC. The management of septal perforations. Plast Reconstr Surg. 1993; 91(2):229–235

[10] Kridel RW, Foda H, Lunde KC. Septal perforation repair with acellular human dermal allograft. Arch Otolaryngol Head Neck Surg. 1998; 124(1):73–78

[11] Woolford TJ, Jones NS. Repair of nasal septal perforations using local mucosal flaps and a composite cartilage graft. J Laryngol Otol. 2001; 115(1):22–25

[12] Ambro BT, Zimmerman J, Rosenthal M, Pribitkin EA. Nasal septal perforation repair with porcine small intestinal submucosa. Arch Facial Plast Surg. 2003; 5(6):528–529

[13] Romo T, III, Jablonski RD, Shapiro AL, McCormick SA. Long-term nasal mucosal tissue expansion use in repair of large nasoseptal perforations. Arch Otolaryngol Head Neck Surg. 1995; 121(3):327–331

[14] Murrell GL, Karakla DW, Messa A. Free flap repair of septal perforation. Plast Reconstr Surg. 1998; 102(3):818–821

[15] Paloma V, Samper A, Cervera-Paz FJ. Surgical technique for reconstruction of the nasal septum: the pericranial flap. Head Neck. 2000; 22(1):90–94

[16] Pribaz J, Stephens W, Crespo L, Gifford G. A new intraoral flap: facial artery musculomucosal (FAMM) flap. Plast Reconstr Surg. 1992; 90 (3):421–429

[17] Ayad T, Kolb F, De Monès E, Mamelle G, Tan HK, Temam S. [The musculo-mucosal facial artery flap: harvesting technique and indications] [in French]. Ann Chir Plast Esthet. 2008; 53(6):487–494

[18] Pinar YA, Bilge O, Govsa F. Anatomic study of the blood supply of perioral region. Clin Anat. 2005; 18(5):330–339

[19] Standring S. Gray's Anatomy—The Anatomical Basis of Clinical Practice. 39th ed. Edinburgh, UK: Elsevier, Churchill Livingstone; 2005: 509–510

[20] Rouviere H, Delmas A. Anatomie humaine descriptive, topographique et fonctionnelle. Tome 1: tête et cou. 15th ed. Paris, France: Masson; 2002

[21] Nakajima H, Imanishi N, Aiso S. Facial artery in the upper lip and nose: anatomy and a clinical application. Plast Reconstr Surg. 2002; 109(3):855–861, discussion 862–863

[22] Lohn JW, Penn JW, Norton J, Butler PE. The course and variation of the facial artery and vein: implications for facial transplantation and facial surgery. Ann Plast Surg. 2011; 67(2):184–188

[23] Zhao Z, Li S, Xu J, et al. Color Doppler flow imaging of the facial artery and vein. Plast Reconstr Surg. 2000; 106(6):1249–1253

[24] Dupoirieux L, Plane L, Gard C, Penneau M. Anatomical basis and results of the facial artery musculomucosal flap for oral reconstruction. Br J Oral Maxillofac Surg. 1999; 37(1):25–28

[25] **Ayad T, Xie L. Facial artery musculomucosal flap in head and neck reconstruction: a systematic review. Head Neck. 2015; 37(9):1375–1386**

[26] Ayad T, Kolb F, De Monés E, Mamelle G, Temam S. Reconstruction of floor of mouth defects by the facial artery musculo-mucosal flap following cancer ablation. Head Neck. 2008; 30(4):437–445

[27] Massarelli O, Gobbi R, Soma D, Tullio A. The folded tunnelized-facial artery myomucosal island flap: a new technique for total soft palate reconstruction. J Oral Maxillofac Surg. 2013; 71(1):192–198

[28] O'Leary P, Bundgaard T. Good results in patients with defects after intraoral tumour excision using facial artery musculo-mucosal flap. Dan Med Bull. 2011; 58(5):A4264

[29] Park C, Lineaweaver WC, Buncke HJ. New perioral arterial flaps: anatomic study and clinical application. Plast Reconstr Surg. 1994; 94(2): 268–276

[30] Céruse P, Ramade A, Dubreuil C, Disant F. [The myo-mucosal buccinator island flap: indications and limits for the reconstruction of deficits of the buccal cavity of the oropharynx] [in French]. J Otolaryngol. 2006; 35(6):404–407

Chapter 19
"Slide and Patch" Technique

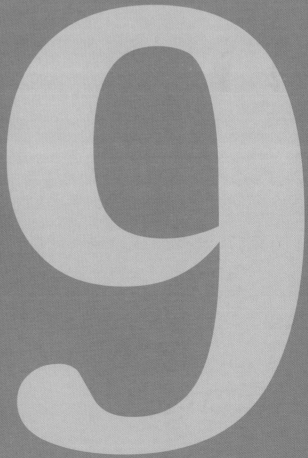

19 "Slide and Patch" Technique

Michele Cassano

Summary

The "slide and patch" technique is so-called because it combines a mucoperiosteal free graft of the inferior turbinate with a mucosal rotational or advancement flap from nasal septum. In fact, the technique implies a "slide" of a mucoperichondrial or mucoperiosteal flap from the septum and a "patch" made by a mucoperiosteal graft harvested from inferior turbinate.

This approach is indicated when the patient has a rounded or oval perforation with larger diameter between 5 and 30 mm. Perforation whose diameter is smaller than 5 mm can be repaired with just a mucoperiosteal graft from inferior turbinate (with a notable time saving). If the perforation is larger than 30 mm, the results cannot be so good because the width of the mucoperiosteal graft could be not so large to cover the defect with a sufficient amount of tissue covered (in an underlay fashion) by the mucosa around the defect. Moreover, it is possible that larger defects cannot leave a sufficient amount of normal mucosa to allow the rotation or the advancement of an adequate flap.

19.1 Indications

- This approach is indicated when the patient has a rounded or oval perforation with larger diameter between 5 and 30 mm.
- Patients with septal perforation and no past history of inferior turbinectomy.

19.2 Surgical Steps

The "slide and patch" technique[1] involves the following surgical steps:

1. The surgery is performed under general anesthesia with the patient in supine position with the head rotated 30 degrees toward the first surgeon and by an endoscopic approach using a 4-mm 30-degree rigid endoscope.
2. Before surgery, two neurosurgical cottonoid pads with naphazoline for each nostril are applied to make a decongestant effect.
3. The nasal mucosa from anterior septum to the nasal floor and till perforation borders is bilaterally infiltrated with lidocaine and 1% adrenaline solution (1:100,000).
4. The perforation margins are then bilaterally trimmed and widely detached all around the perforation from the underlying cartilage or bone by a sickle knife to achieve a "refreshening of the edge" (▶ Fig. 19.1). It is important to elevate bilaterally an area of mucoperiosteum or mucoperichondrium of at least 1 cm all around the perforation.
5. Through a hemitransfixion incision, mucoperichondrial and mucoperiosteal layers are extensively elevated on one side of the nasal septum, from the inferior edge of quadrilateral cartilage up to the choana, nasal floor, and 1 cm from the nasal roof (▶ Fig. 19.2).
6. On the other side, in oval perforation with horizontal major diameter, a horizontal incision as long as the perforation major diameter is performed by a sickle

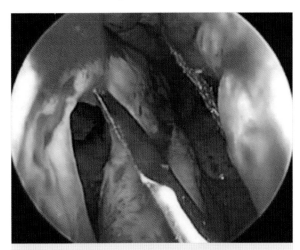

Fig. 19.1 The perforation margins are bilaterally trimmed and widely dissected all around the perforation from the underlying cartilage or bone by a sickle knife.

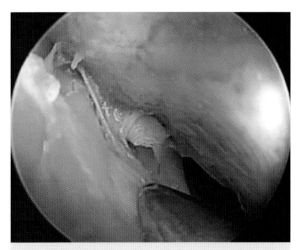

Fig. 19.2 Through a hemitransfix incision, mucoperichondrial and mucoperiosteal layers are extensively elevated on one side of the nasal septum.

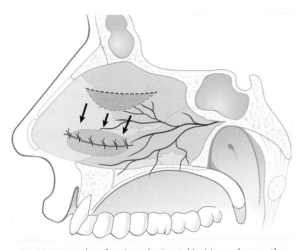

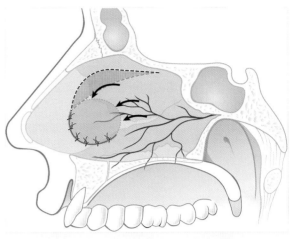

Fig. 19.3 In oval perforation a horizontal incision as long as the perforation major diameter is performed by a sickle knife on nasal mucosa 1 cm to the dorsal border of septal cartilage. The mucoperichondrial flap is then elevated from the perforation margin up to the incision and the flap is transposed downward and the borders of the perforation are sutured together with a 3–0 Vicryl suture.

Fig. 19.4 In rounded perforations, a rotation/advancement mucoperiosteal flap based on the nasal-septal artery is designed and rotated to reach the inferior border of the perforation.

knife on nasal mucosa 1 cm to the dorsal border of septal cartilage. The mucoperichondrial flap is then elevated from the perforation margin up to the incision. The flap is thus transposed downward and the borders of the perforation are sutured together with a 3–0 Vicryl suture (▶ Fig. 19.3).

7. In the case of rounded perforations, a rotation/advancement mucoperiosteal flap is designed by a rounded incision based posteriorly on the nasal-septal artery and elevated up to 1 cm from the choana (▶ Fig. 19.4). Also, in this case the flap is rotated to reach the inferior border of the perforation and sutured with a 3–0 Vicryl suture (▶ Fig. 19.5).

8. In both cases the flap should advance to cover the perforation without tension. The septal cartilage of the area where the flap has been prepared is left uncovered.

9. A mucoperiosteal graft is harvested from the inferior turbinate by an endoscopic turbinoplasty following Marks' technique.[2] In particular, after injecting 2 to 3 mL of solution containing 1% Carbocaine with 1:80,000 epinephrine on inferior turbinate mucosa, over the bone, an incision on the head of the inferior turbinate with a number 15 blade along the inferior edge of the turbinate is performed. The mucoperiosteum of the nasal side of the turbinate is thus separated by a suction elevator from the underlying bone. The turbinate bone with attached lateral mucosa is then removed by endoscopic scissors till the tail of the turbinate; the residual bone can be outfractured to reduce the angle between the turbinate and lateral nasal wall. Finally the mucosa of the nasal side

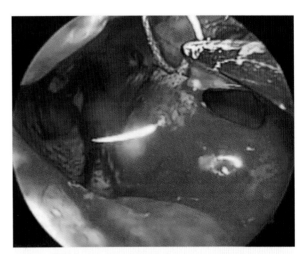

Fig. 19.5 The flap is sutured to the borders of the perforation by a 3–0 Vicryl suture.

(previously elevated) is flipped over to cover the exposed area.

10. The removed part of the inferior turbinate (▶ Fig. 19.6) is therefore used to harvest the graft by separating the mucoperiosteum (lateral mucosa of the inferior turbinate) from the underlying bone (▶ Fig. 19.7). The mucoperiosteal graft is trimmed to size (minimum 1 cm of diameter larger than the perforation).

11. The mucoperiosteal graft is then inserted through the hemitransfix incision in the tunnel between the septal cartilage and elevated septal mucoperichondrial flap (▶ Fig. 19.8).

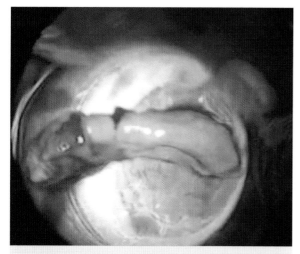

Fig. 19.6 The lateral part of inferior turbinate has been removed by an endoscopic turbinoplasty.

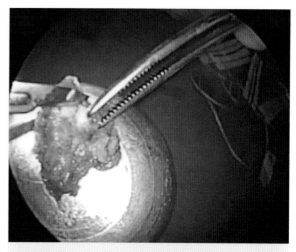

Fig. 19.7 The removed part of the inferior turbinate is therefore used to harvest the graft by separating the mucoperiosteum from the underlying bone. The mucoperiosteal flap is trimmed to size (minimum 1 cm of diameter larger than the perforation).

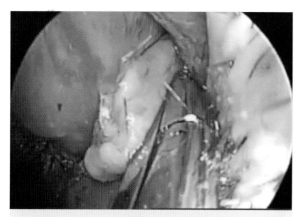

Fig. 19.8 The mucoperiosteal flap is inserted through the hemitransfix incision in the tunnel between the septal cartilage and the elevated septal mucoperichondrial flap.

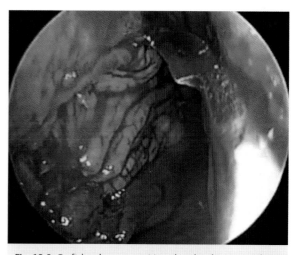

Fig. 19.9 Graft borders are positioned under the previously elevated perforation borders in underlay fashion.

12. Graft borders are positioned under the previously elevated perforation borders in underlay fashion for minimum 5 mm all around (▸ Fig. 19.9).
13. At the end of this step, no one area of the perforation has to be uncovered (▸ Fig. 19.10).
14. A Gelfoam sheet can be positioned over the graft to protect it in the healing process.
15. Silastic sheets, designed to cover nasal septum from 1 cm below the septal roof up to the nasal floor, are inserted bilaterally and fixed anteriorly and posteriorly by a 2–0 silk "U" suture.
16. Nasal packing is rarely necessary if careful control of bleeding and cauterization of bleeding points is performed under endoscopic vision before ending surgery.[3]

17. Antibiotic therapy is prescribed with amoxicillin and clavulanic acid (1 g twice a day orally) and tranexamic acid (1 fL twice a day orally) starting the night of the surgery.
18. Starting the next day, nasal lavages are frequently performed with lukewarm sterile saline solution.
19. The patients can be discharged on the first postoperative day, if nasal packing has not been applied and if there is not an active nasal bleeding.
20. A postoperative checkup is performed once a week, and for the first 2 weeks in particular this is to remove the scabs or clots and evaluate the postoperative healing.
21. Silastic sheets are removed at about 3 weeks postoperatively.

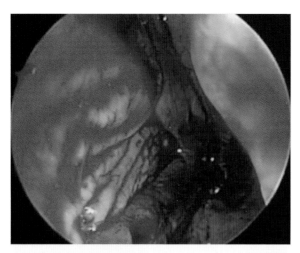

Fig. 19.10 The result at the end of surgery before positioning the Silastic sheets.

22. Subsequent checkups are performed weekly until the full integrity of the mucosa is restored. It is important to avoid aspiration and pay particular attention to removing the scabs and clots that lie on the flap or on the graft because those can displace the graft. It is better to let the nasal lavages removing the scabs and clots and to gently remove them with a forceps starting from 1 month postoperatively

19.3 Advantages and Disadvantages

This technique provides many advantages: first, the use of a flap of native septal tissue with the advantage of the rich vascular supply and the proximity to the defect. In fact, in case of rotational flap, the nasal-septal artery (from sphenopalatine artery) supplies the flap, whereas in case of advancement flap both nasal-septal artery and septal branch of anterior ethmoidal artery supply the flap.

Another advantage can be the use of autologous nasal mucosa grafts because it enables to completely maintain the normal nasal physiology integrating perfectly with the septal nasal mucosa. Moreover, the graft is relatively easy to harvest without donor site morbidity. In fact, Marks' turbinoplasty is a simple procedure that allows the patient to improve nasal breathing, without altering the shape and function of the inferior turbinate because the removed part is just the meatal part of the turbinate with complete saving of respiratory mucosa.[2] Techniques that involve the harvesting of the graft from other donor sites (temporalis fascia, fascia lata, etc.) obviously cause a double donor site morbidity.[4,5,6,7,8]

Finally "slide and patch " technique provide a two-layer repair of nasal-septal defect in which the mucoperiosteal graft not only serves as a scaffold for the migration of respiratory mucosa but also provides a second layer of defense. Although the use of a unilateral flap is considered insufficient by some authors[9] and other authors reported that the repair with bilateral flaps is the most important factor for successful closure,[10,11] the use of a single flap associated with a graft showed a percentage of success as high as or, in some cases, higher than those reported in studies in which bilateral flaps and interposition graft were used.[1] Obviously the preparation of a single flap implies a shortening of the operation time compared to bilateral flap techniques.

The only disadvantage of this technique is that it requires a great deal of training and skill in endoscopic nasal surgery because endoscopic suturing and harvesting the flap is not a skill for beginners and requires a prolonged time also in experienced hands.

19.4 Case Example

A 44-year-old man came to the Department of Otorhinolaryngology of the University of Foggia, complaining of crusting and recurrent epistaxis since 2 years after a septoplasty performed in another hospital.

The nasal endoscopy revealed a 2.3-cm diameter rounded perforation 2 cm posteriorly to nasal nostrils and abundant crusting all around the perforation.

The perforation was repaired by a "slide and patch" technique using a rotation/advancement mucoperiosteal flap based posteriorly on the nasal-septal artery and elevated up to 1 cm from the choana in the right side and a mucoperiosteal graft in the left side.

No complication occurred during surgery and the patient was discharged 2 days after surgery without packing. After 3 weeks the Silastic sheets were removed revealing a perfect healing of the graft and of the flap.

After 1 month postoperatively the patient came back to the hospital for appearance of nasal obstruction in left nasal fossa. A nasal endoscopy revealed a hypertrophy of the graft tissue with increasing of nasal resistances at rhinomanometry (3.5 Pa/cm^3/s at 150 Pa). A nasal spray with furoate mometasone was suggested once a day for 3 month to reduce the hypertrophy, but the patient did not resolve the problem. Therefore 6 months after the first operation, radiofrequencies ($75°C$, 250 J) were applied on the hypertrophied graft in local anesthesia by a Somnus S2 generator (Gyrus ENT LLC). After 1 month the patient resolved his nasal obstruction with improvement of rhinomanometric resistances (1.1 Pa/cm^3/s).

19.5 Tips and Tricks

The "slide and patch" technique, as most of the endoscopic techniques of septal perforation repair, requires a wide detachment of the mucoperichondrium and mucoperiosteum of both sides of the septum and all around the perforation. This step is very important because it allows to rotate and advance the flaps without tension and to easily allocate the graft in underlay fashion.

The most difficult step in this technique is the endoscopic suture of the flap. We suggest performing the suture introducing endoscopically the needle till reaching the flap and taking it at 2 mm from the flap border. Then the other border can be joining at the same time or after the needle has come out from the first border. In some case we can catch again the needle in the opposite nasal fossa and then reenter in the side of the flap catching the other margin. When the needle has joined both margins, it can be taken out from the nose and the knot is performed outside. At this moment the second surgeon will hold one end of the thread and the first surgeon will drive endoscopically the other end into the nose, till tightening the knot. This procedure must be repeated for minimum two times to guarantee the stability of the knot.

Another important tip is to harvest a large mucoperiosteal graft that can be widely positioned under the perforation borders to avoid that the retraction of the graft during the healing process will uncover a part of perforation.

Moreover, it is very important to thin the graft, eventually flattening it in a Cottle cartilage crusher. This trick will avoid the bulging of the graft in the nasal fossa with consequent nasal obstruction (see illustrative case).

When we are positioning the graft, to avoid it to slip posteriorly, a good trick could be to fix the anterior margin of the graft to the septum with a 3–0 Vicryl. In this way we can put the graft underlay without leaving an anterior area uncovered.

Another tip that we want to suggest is to avoid tightening too much the Silastic sheets and packing patients because an excessive pressure on the flaps can reduce the vascularization and delay or alter the healing process.

A particular caution must be taken during the first postoperative checkups because a too intense aspiration can dislocate the graft or can remove the fibrin between the flap and the perforation margins, altering the healing process.

19.6 Complications and Technical Solutions

See ▶ Table 19.1 to evaluate the points of difficulty and possible technical solutions.

19.7 Conclusion

The endoscopic "slide and patch" technique has shown optimal results in nasal-septal perforation repair. Although this approach requires a great deal of training and skill in endoscopic nasal surgery, it has the advantage of not requiring graft from outside the nose (avoiding donor site morbidity) and of shortening the operation time, with repair rates similar to techniques with bilateral flaps.

Table 19.1 Complications and technical solutions

Complications	Technical solutions
An important bleeding during surgery could make difficult the harvesting of the flaps	Positioning of neurosurgical cottonoid pads with naphazoline before surgery for 5–10 min and accurate infiltration of septal mucosa and perforation borders with lidocaine and 1% adrenaline solution (100,000:1)
The flap does not completely cover the defect on one side of the septal perforation	Do not plan this surgery when you do not have an area of mucosa over the defect as large as the perforation
The flap advances or rotates with tension	Mucoperichondrial and mucoperiosteal layers must be extensively elevated from the nasal floor up to 1 cm from the nasal roof and posteriorly up to the choana, esp. in rotational flaps
Suturing the flap to the perforation borders	Insert the needle endoscopically taking both borders separately, then come out with the needle; make the knot outside and push it endoscopically into the nose again.
Positioning the graft in underlay fashion without leaving uncovered part of the perforation	Harvest a sufficiently large mucoperiosteal graft (1 cm larger than perforation diameter) and elevate an area of mucoperiosteum or mucoperichondrium of at least 1 cm all around the perforation
The graft does not easily enter through the mucoperichondrial tunnel	A large hemitransfix incision must be performed. Mucoperichondrial and mucoperiosteal layers must be extensively elevated on that side of the nasal septum, from the inferior edge of quadrilateral cartilage up to the choana, nasal floor and 1 cm from the nasal roof
Positioning of the Silastic sheets without dislocating the graft	Try to fix the Silastic sheet anteriorly in the vestibular area (before the anterior margin of the graft and posteriorly in the lower part of nasal septum where native mucosa is present)

References

[1] Cassano M. Endoscopic repair of nasal septal perforation with "slide and patch" technique. Otolaryngol Head Neck Surg. 2014; 151(1): 176–178

[2] Marks S. Endoscopic inferior turbinoplasty. Am J Rhinol. 1998; 12(6): 405–407

[3] Cassano M, Longo M, Fiocca-Matthews E, Del Giudice AM. Endoscopic intraoperative control of epistaxis in nasal surgery. Auris Nasus Larynx. 2010; 37(2):178–184

[4] Chen FH, Rui X, Deng J, Wen YH, Xu G, Shi JB. Endoscopic sandwich technique for moderate nasal septal perforations. Laryngoscope. 2012; 122(11):2367–2372

[5] Yenigun A, Meric A, Verim A, Ozucer B, Yasar H, Ozkul MH. Septal perforation repair: mucosal regeneration technique. Eur Arch Otorhinolaryngol. 2012; 269(12):2505–2510

[6] Taskin U, Yigit O, Sisman SA. Septal perforation repairing with combination of mucosal flaps and auricular interpositional grafts in revision patients. Otolaryngol Head Neck Surg. 2011; 145(5): 828–832

[7] Kaya E, Cingi C, Olgun Y, Soken H, Pinarbasli Ö. Three layer interlocking: a novel technique for repairing a nasal septum perforation. Ann Otol Rhinol Laryngol. 2015; 124(3):212–215

[8] Bank J, Beederman M, Naclerio RM, Gottlieb LJ. Prelaminated fascia lata free flap for large nasal septal defect reconstruction. J Plast Reconstr Aesthet Surg. 2014; 67(10):1440–1443

[9] Kridel RW. Considerations in the etiology, treatment, and repair of septal perforations. Facial Plast Surg Clin North Am. 2004; 12(4): 435–450, vi

[10] Kim SW, Rhee CS. Nasal septal perforation repair: predictive factors and systematic review of the literature. Curr Opin Otolaryngol Head Neck Surg. 2012; 20(1):58–65

[11] Moon IJ, Kim SW, Han DH, et al. Predictive factors for the outcome of nasal septal perforation repair. Auris Nasus Larynx. 2011; 38(1): 52–57

Chapter 20

Backward Extraction-Reposition Technique of Quadrangular Cartilage

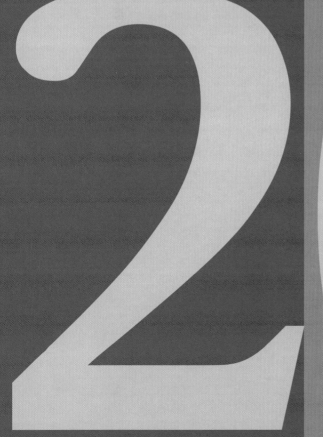
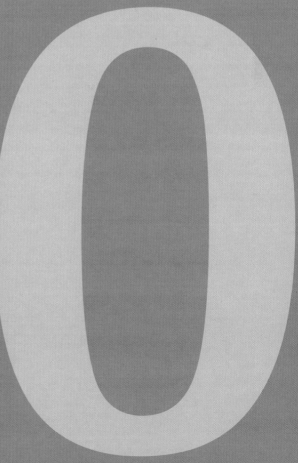

20 Backward Extraction-Reposition Technique of Quadrangular Cartilage

Ignazio Tasca, Giacomo Ceroni Compadretti

Summary

Surgical repair of septal perforations represents a complex technical challenge for the surgeon. Many different surgical techniques have been proposed for the closure of septal perforations, but there is no standard protocol universally accepted. The Cottle technique is a viable procedure for the closure of small- and middle-sized perforations. We here present our experience, using the Cottle technique with the backward extraction-reposition of nasal septum and inverted sliding flap suture technique. A fundamental prognostic indicator of successful surgery is the amount of septal structures remaining within the rest of the septum. An important surgical success factor is the surgeon's experience and skill. Correction of concomitant nasal deformities improves functional results and patient satisfaction; the reduction in flow turbulences avoids drying of the mucosa and consequently the risk of reperforation.

20.1 Indication

- Symptomatic small- to medium-sized perforation

20.2 Surgical Anatomy and Operative Implications

Nasal septal perforations (NSPs) are anatomical defects of nasal septum caused by the necrosis of the cartilage and/or bone tissues and their mucous covering. Perforations are classically distinguished according to their etiopathogenic factors, size, and location.[1,2,3] Size and location must be considered because they determine the choice of the reconstructive procedure and consequently the closure rate success. For this purpose, some basics of anatomy should be considered by the surgeon to discriminate the amount and the type of tissue defect, whereas the knowledge of septal vascularization is essential for the planning of the endonasal flaps.

The nasal septum divides the nose into two cavities. The bony components of the septum include the nasal crest of the palatine bone, nasal crest of the maxilla and premaxilla, vomer, perpendicular plate of the ethmoid, nasal crest of the frontal bone, and spine of the paired nasal bones. The anterior septum is composed of the quadrilateral cartilage and joins the free edges of the aforementioned bones. The anterior superior margin of

the quadrangular cartilage joins, at its extreme cephalic, with the caudal end of the median suture of nasal bones contributing, together with the ethmoid perpendicular plate and the upper lateral cartilages, gives the support of the nasal vault. The anterior superior angle of the septal cartilage, defined as *septal angle*, constitutes an important surgical point. The septal angle is located immediately above the lower lateral cartilages in the *supratip* area. The loss of cartilaginous support in this area can cause the collapse of the mid-nasal vault. The caudal margin goes from lobule to the nasal spine, contracting relationships with the membranous septum. The caudal edge presents an intermediate angle and a posterior angle just above the nasal spine.

The osteocartilaginous skeleton is covered by periosteum and perichondrium, which are highly vascularized. The arterial blood supply consists of terminals from the external and internal carotid systems.[4] The sphenopalatine artery, terminal branch of the internal maxillary artery (external carotid artery), gives rise to outer branches such as the artery of the middle turbinate and the artery of the inferior turbinate, and also internal branches such as the septal artery that gives rise to the artery of the upper turbinate and septal arteries.

All these arteries anastomose with the ethmoid arteries. The underseptal artery, branch of the facial artery, runs along the nasal vestibule region and the lower anterior septal cartilage. The anterior ethmoid artery, branch of the ophthalmic artery (internal carotid), gives rise to two branches: an internal nasal and external nasal branches, which supply the frontal sinuses and ethmoid cells. The internal and external posterior ethmoidal arteries have anastomose with the anterior ethmoidal artery at the level of the turbinates and with the sphenopalatine artery in the upper part of the septum.

20.3 Patient Selection

Surgical repair of septal perforations represents a complex technical challenge for the surgeon. The principal aims of the surgery are to repair the mucous and also to reestablish the function and physiology of the nose.[5] Many different surgical techniques have been proposed for the closure of septal perforations, but there is no standard protocol universally accepted.[6,7,8,9,10] This multitude of different techniques suggests that there is no better procedure than another, but several factors play a role in both decision making of surgical planning and treatment success.[11] A fundamental prognostic indicator of successful surgery is the amount of septal structures remaining within the rest of the septum. An important surgical success factor is the surgeon's experience and skill. Another critical factor is the adequate view of the operative field, and thus the collaboration of the anesthesiologist is essential to achieve an effective haemostasis. All the techniques are also variably associated with a number of different grafts, both autologous and heterologous, to obtain a safer closure.[12,13] More recently, some authors have developed the endoscopic approach to improve visualization without performing an excessive dissection.[14,15,16,17,18]

In case of small- to medium-sized perforation, the endonasal approach is the treatment of choice. The backward extraction-reposition technique allows the defects of cartilage and mucoperichondral-mucoperiosteal coating to be situated on two different levels, making safer the strength of the suture of the flap.[19] A further safe point is also provided by the inverted sliding flap suture (▶ Fig. 20.1). This asymmetric movement of flaps enables a nonopposing suture line and a better mucoperichondral blood supply to the repositioned graft.[20] The endonasal approach, compared with open techniques, enables a small incision, without sacrificing tissues or structures for improving the exposition. We must consider that any incision is bounded to undergo some degree of contraction after surgery, so it is more convenient to perform the lowest number of incisions, above all in this type of surgery. Furthermore, many perforation repair

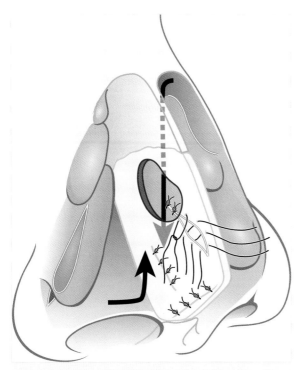

Fig. 20.1 Schematic representation of the backward extraction-reposition technique of the quadrangular cartilage with inverted sliding flap suture.

procedures often require the use of interpositional autografts between the repaired flaps and they are consequently accompanied by donor site morbidity. Contrarily, this technique, by repositioning the remaining nasal septum, does not require further supporting implants and that way allows the perforation to be closed without associated morbidity.

20.4 Surgical Steps

1. The septum is achieved by the endonasal approach through the classic hemitransfixion incision. The caudal margin of the septal cartilage should be completely exposed using suction dissector with careful movements.
2. Once the caudal margin is exposed, the surgeon begins creating the anterior tunnels along the subperichondral avascular plane. Dissection must be performed carefully around the perforation without opening it.
3. Subperiosteal inferior tunnels are then created along the floor of the nasal cavities after exposing the nasal spine, the anterior-inferior septal angle, and the medial portion of the inferior margin of the pyriform aperture.
4. Next, the four tunnels are joined and the septal space is exposed, allowing a general view of the whole septum and its bony framework.
5. Only at this moment the perforation is opened by a mucosal incision to separate the two nasal cavities. With the aid of a nasal speculum, the entire septum can be visualized from vault to floor.
6. After performing the subtriangular chondrotomy and posterior osteotomy, the residual septum is extracted leaving only a small 3-mm strip of cartilage close to the keystone area.
7. Next, an incision is made in the floor of the nasal cavity at the inferior turbinate insertion. In the contralateral nasal cavity an incision is made in the same direction at the roof. When the flaps have been prepared, it is necessary to slide asymmetrically in a cranial direction in one nasal cavity, and in a caudal direction, in the contralateral cavity.
8. The closure of the mucosal perforation is achieved by using a 4–0 Polysorb braided absorbable suture. The flap made from the nasal floor is an axial flap, based on the branches of the superior labial artery. Being a mucoperiosteal flap, it is suitable for the purpose because it is quite thick and strong. It can be enlarged according to need, and it has a potential size of 2.5 × 4 cm in most patients.
9. Once the mucosal perforation is closed in both sides, a soft nasal packing is placed into the nasal cavities and pushed posteriorly toward the nasopharynx and up to the attic.

10. On a back table, the septum is reconstructed to fill the defect and create a regular graft to be repositioned.

11. Cartilage graft fixation is accomplished by a three-point suture using a 2–0 Safil polyglicolic acid braided absorbable suture with 60-mm straight needle.

12. The nasal packing is maintained for 2 days to ensure that the flap adheres and to prevent septal hematoma and displacement of the inserted fragments. Fluoroplastic nasal splints are also positioned into the nasal cavities. They remain to guide healings and then removed after 15 days.

13. In the large perforations associated with external deformities of the nose, the provision of intranasal tissue to close the perforation can be obtained with methods of downward displacement of the pyramid: the push-down and the let-down. The push-down is used to correct the bony and cartilaginous hump.[21] It requires to perform the basal and transverse osteotomy. When the osteocartilaginous deformity occurs on a prominent pyramid above all in the cartilaginous vault, let-down technique can be implemented. Compared to the push-down that drops the nasal pyramid in the nasal cavity, the let-down lowers the pyramid relative to the plane of the face without determining volume inside the nasal cavity. It provides for a double basal osteotomy for the removal of a bony triangle, symmetric or asymmetric according to the needs, and the transverse osteotomy that allows the lowering of the pyramid downward (Video 20.1).

20.5 Complications and Technical Solutions

▶ Table 20.1 discusses points of difficulty and technical solutions.

Table 20.1 Complications and technical solutions

Complication	Technical solution
Possible enlargement of the mucosal perforation during the dissection	Incision of the mucosa around the perforation only at the end of the dissection
Nasal dorsal collapse and keystone area destabilization	Preserve a 0.3-mm dorsal cartilaginous without cutting the upper lateral cartilages Make a careful graft fixation
Closure of the mucosal perforation without tension	Move wide flaps by making a large dissection toward the insertion of the inferior turbinate and up to the nasal vault

20.6 Case Examples

20.6.1 Case 1

A 32-year-old man presented complaining of whistling and nasal obstruction for many years. The patient tried medical therapy without success. He reported clinical history of nasal chemical or electrical cauterization for epistaxis during childhood. In anterior rhinoscopy, he presented a small-sized perforation of the anterior nasal septum (▶ Fig. 20.2). After septum extraction, a further undiagnosed cartilaginous defect appeared posteriorly (▶ Fig. 20.3). The patient was successfully operated by the backward extraction-reposition of nasal septum technique. At 1-year follow-up the nasal septum was definitely restored, the patient reported an adequate nasal respiration, and he was satisfied with the results (▶ Fig. 20.4).

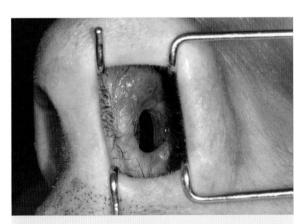

Fig. 20.2 Rhinoscopic view of the left nasal cavity showing a small-sized and circularly shaped perforation of anterior nasal septum.

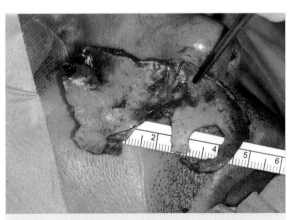

Fig. 20.3 Intraoperative view of the removed nasal septum showing an additional posterior defect of the cartilage not previously diagnosable.

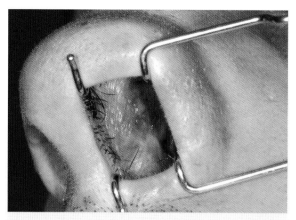

Fig. 20.4 Rhinoscopic view of the left nasal cavity at 1-year follow-up showing a completely restored nasal septum with closed perforation.

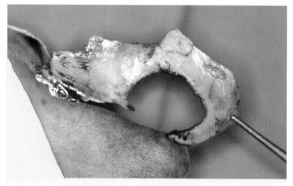

Fig. 20.6 Intraoperative view of the extracted septum consisting of the vomer and the remnants of the quadrangular cartilage.

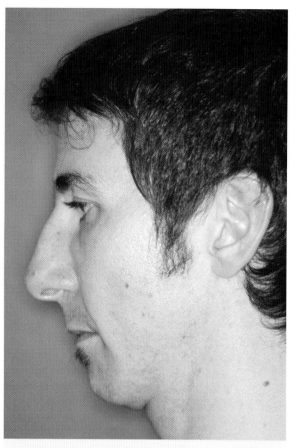

Fig. 20.5 Preoperative left lateral view. The dorsum profile is deformed by an osteocartilaginous hump.

20.6.2 Case 2

A 38-year-old man was cocaine addict for many years. The patient reported symptoms of nasal obstruction with crusting. He was very symptomatic despite nasal irrigations and ointment applications. He was diagnosed with an anterior medium-sized NSP with external pyramid deformity due to the presence of a hump of the nasal dorsum (▶ Fig. 20.5). He was treated by backward extraction-reposition of nasal septum technique associated with push-down procedure (▶ Fig. 20.6, ▶ Fig. 20.7). After 1-year follow-up the patient reported normal nasal breathing with closed perforation and presented a regular nasal profile (▶ Fig. 20.8). In this case the correction of the external deformity of the pyramid allowed a greater amount of tissue to close the perforation and also achieved an aesthetical improvement.

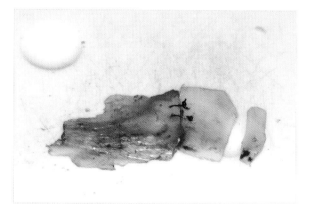

Fig. 20.7 Back table view of the extracorporeal reconstruction of the neo-septum.

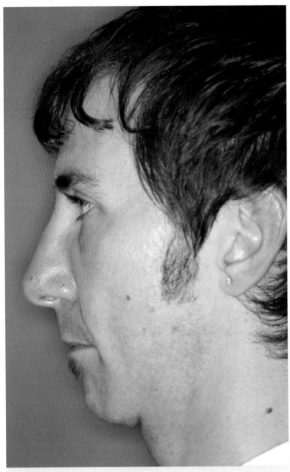

Fig. 20.8 Postoperative left lateral view at 1 year follow-up. It can be appreciated as normalization of the dorsal profile.

20.7 Tips and Tricks

- Preliminary infiltration of lidocaine with adrenaline on subperichondral and subperiosteal dissection is essential to get a minimal intraoperative bleeding.
- Do the incision of the mucosa around the perforation only at the end of the dissection maneuvers to prevent enlargements of the defect during flap elevation.
- Correction of concomitant nasal deformities improves functional results and patient satisfaction; the reduction in flow turbulences avoids drying of the mucosa and consequently the risk of re-perforation.
- Accurate reconstruction and making suture without tension of the septal skeleton prevent from reperforation.

- Make soft nasal packing is important to avoid ischemia of the flaps providing good sustenance to the reconstructed septum.
- Splint application serves as guidance during the healing process.

References

[1] Kridel RW. Septal perforation repair. Otolaryngol Clin North Am. 1999; 32(4):695–724

[2] Brain DJ. Septo-rhinoplasty: the closure of septal perforations. J Laryngol Otol. 1980; 94(5):495–505

[3] Younger R, Blokmanis A. Nasal septal perforations. J Otolaryngol. 1985; 14(2):125–131

[4] Chiu T, Dunn JS. An anatomical study of the arteries of the anterior nasal septum. Otolaryngol Head Neck Surg. 2006; 134(1):33–36

[5] Kuriloff DB. Nasal septal perforations and nasal obstruction. Otolaryngol Clin North Am. 1989; 22(2):333–350

[6] Fairbanks DN. Closure of nasal septal perforations. Arch Otolaryngol. 1980; 106(8):509–513

[7] Kridel RWH, Appling WD, Wright WK. Septal perforation closure utilizing the external septorhinoplasty approach. Arch Otolaryngol Head Neck Surg. 1986; 112(2):168–172

[8] Romo T, III, Foster CA, Korovin GS, Sachs ME. Repair of nasal septal perforation utilizing the midface degloving technique. Arch Otolaryngol Head Neck Surg. 1988; 114(7):739–742

[9] Karlan MS, Ossoff RH, Sisson GA. A compendium of intranasal flaps. Laryngoscope. 1982; 92(7 Pt 1):774–782

[10] Goh AY, Hussain SS. Different surgical treatments for nasal septal perforation and their outcomes. J Laryngol Otol. 2007; 121(5):419–426

[11] Kim SW, Rhee CS. Nasal septal perforation repair: predictive factors and systematic review of the literature. Curr Opin Otolaryngol Head Neck Surg. 2012; 20(1):58–65

[12] Stoor P, Grénman R. Bioactive glass and turbinate flaps in the repair of nasal septal perforations. Ann Otol Rhinol Laryngol. 2004; 113(8):655–661

[13] Ambro BT, Zimmerman J, Rosenthal M, Pribitkin EA. Nasal septal perforation repair with porcine small intestinal submucosa. Arch Facial Plast Surg. 2003; 5(6):528–529

[14] Friedman M, Ibrahim H, Ramakrishnan V. Inferior turbinate flap for repair of nasal septal perforation. Laryngoscope. 2003; 113(8):1425–1428

[15] Hier MP, Yoskovitch A, Panje WR. Endoscopic repair of a nasal septal perforation. J Otolaryngol. 2002; 31(5):323–326

[16] Presutti L, Alicandri-Ciufelli M, Marchioni D, Ghidini A, Villari D. Surgery of septal perforations. Plast Reconstr Surg. 2008; 122(1):22e–23e

[17] Castelnuovo P, Ferreli F, Khodaei I, Palma P. Anterior ethmoidal artery septal flap for the management of septal perforation. Arch Facial Plast Surg. 2011; 13(6):411–414

[18] Giacomini PG, Ferraro S, Di Girolamo S, Ottaviani F. Large nasal septal perforation repair by closed endoscopically assisted approach. Ann Plast Surg. 2011; 66(6):633–636

[19] Sarandeses-García A, Sulsenti G, López-Amado M, Martínez-Vidal J. Septal perforations closure utilizing the backwards extraction-reposition technique of the quadrangular cartilage. J Laryngol Otol. 1999; 113(8):721–724

[20] Tasca I, Compadretti GC. Closure of nasal septal perforation via endonasal approach. Otolaryngol Head Neck Surg. 2006; 135(6):922–927

[21] Mocella S, Muià F, Giacomini PG, Bertossi D, Residori E, Sgroi S. Innovative technique for large septal perforation repair and radiological evaluation. Acta Otorhinolaryngol Ital. 2013; 33(3):202–214

Chapter 21

Pericranial Flap and Endoscopic Septal Repair

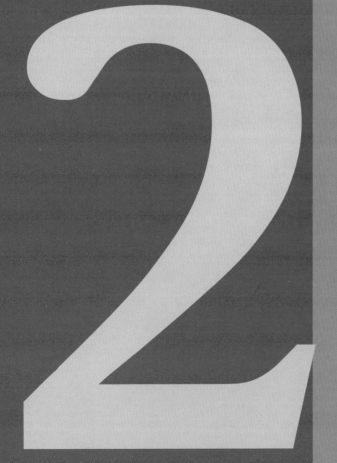

21 Pericranial Flap and Endoscopic Septal Repair

Alfonso Santamaría, Cristobal Langdon, Mauricio López-Chacón, Arturo Cordero Castillo, Isam Alobid

Summary

Large nasal septal perforations have been one of the most difficult nasal defects to reconstruct endoscopically, and no standardized procedure has been accepted as the gold standard. This chapter shows a new endoscopic technique to reconstruct an entire septal perforation. A pericranial flap introduced through the frontal sinus was used to close the perforation.

21.1 Introduction

The pericranial flap has been used for/in many different surgical applications since first described by Wolfe in 1978,[1] due to its excellent vascularity and strength.[2] These applications include closure of the skull-base and orbital defects,[3,4,5] closure of sinus fistula and frontal sinus obliteration,[6,7,8] and support for scalp and skin reconstruction.[9,10,11,12] The use of the pericranial flap in total septum perforation repair surgery is not well documented in the literature. There is one case report[13] that basically outlines the surgical technique but does not study the consequences or the possibility of applying this technique in other patients. There is another article in the literature,[14] which describes a pericranial flap and calvarial bone grafts for septal reconstruction; however, these were not total septal perforations and the technique was used only in cadaver. This surgical method offers us an approach to solving total septum perforation, which has had no effective solution until now.

21.2 Surgical Anatomy

21.2.1 Scalp Anatomy

A good knowledge of the anatomy of the scalp and its layers is essential for a clear understanding of the pericranial flap. The scalp is made up of five tissue layers.
1. Skin.
2. Subcutaneous tissue/connective tissue.
3. Aponeurotic layer/galeal layer includes the frontalis muscle anteriorly, the occipitalis muscle posteriorly, the galea that connects both of them, and the temporoparietal fascia laterally.
4. Loose areolar tissue/subgaleal layer is composed of a central dense collagenous layer surrounded by vascularized areolar tissue. The subgaleal fascia is usually included in pericranial flaps, which are often based beyond the periosteum. The loose areolar tissue is continuous with the temporalis fascia laterally.[2]

5. Pericranium layer is the periosteum of the skull bones and in temporal area joins to the deep temporalis fascia, which overlies the temporalis muscle.

The pericranial flap is formed by the union of the pericranium layer and most of the subgaleal layer[15] (▶ Fig. 21.1).

21.2.2 Blood Supply

The anterior part of the scalp, where you can harvest the pericranial flap, is supplied mainly by two supraorbital (SO) and two supratrochlear (ST) arteries, one of each on each side (see ▶ Fig. 21.1). Both arteries are branches of the ophthalmic artery that is a branch of the internal carotid artery.[16] These arteries enter into the scalp just below the orbital roof and divide either near or above the SO rim into both superficial and deep branches. The superficial branches run through the galea-frontalis layer of the scalp, and the deep branches ascend supplying the pericranium.[17] These arteries anastomose with each other and with the superficial temporal artery laterally, communicating the external and internal carotid systems.[15]

The SO artery, which is the main supply of the pericranial flap, crosses the orbital rim beside the SO notch (or through the foramen), approximately 30 mm from the midline,[18] and divides at this level into superficial and deep branches in 80% of cases.[17] The SO notch is more common than the foramen, being present in approximately 70% of cadaveric specimens.[19]

The ST artery, which is smaller and more medial than the SO artery, emerges through the frontal notch or foramen as part of the neurovascular pedicle, approximately

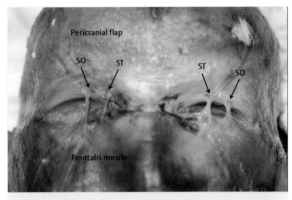

Fig. 21.1 Exits of the supraorbital (SO) and supratrochlear (ST) arteries at the level of the orbital rim. The pericranial flap is composed of the pericranium and the loose areolar tissue; on the other side, the frontalis muscle is covered by the subcutaneous tissue and the skin of the scalp.

22.2 mm from the midline.[19] The division into superficial and deep branches occurs at the level of SO rim or below in 92% of the cases.[17]

Although the division of the SO and ST arteries into superficial and deep branches occurs in most cases at the level of the orbital rim or below, in some cases it occurs above that level. Therefore, it is recommended avoiding extending the separation of the pericranial flap from the galea-frontalis muscle layer into the 10 mm above the orbital rim, to prevent injury to the vascular supply.[17]

21.2.3 Sensory Innervation to Scalp

The sensory innervation of the scalp comes from the SO and the ST nerves. Both are branches of the ophthalmic division of the trigeminal nerve, which divides within the orbit to give rise to these branches. Both of them usually emerge from the superior orbital rim with the arteries of the same name, the SO and the ST arteries, respectively. The ST branch is a small nerve that supplies the anterior midline forehead to the hairline. The SO nerve divides into a superficial branch and a deep branch, and provides the most of sensation in the scalp, from the forehead to the vertex.[20]

21.3 Indications

It has been well established that intranasal vascularized flaps are the best reconstructive options in small-medium septal perforations. However, these flaps are not always available or not large enough to close a septal perforation. The indications could be summarized as

- Large septal perforations, for example in cases of near total septal perforation after surgery, trauma, or drug abuse.
- Intranasal flaps are not available, for example when vascular supply to intranasal flaps has been compromised.

The use of the pericranial flap would be contraindicated in patients who have suffered previous forehead surgery with likely interruption of the blood supply of the flap or in case of orbital rim fractures.

21.4 Surgical Steps

1. At the beginning of surgery, the nasal cavity is decongested with cottonoids impregnated with a solution of adrenalin 0.001% with lidocaine 2%. This aids with hemostasis throughout the surgery. The edges of the septal perforation are refreshed to improve their binding to the flap.[15,21]
2. To introduce the pericranial flap into the nasal cavity, an osteotomy of frontal sinus is needed, which requires a Draf III frontal sinusotomy, as described

previously by Draf in 1991.[22] This procedure involves removal of the interfrontal septum, the superior part of the nasal septum, and the frontal sinus floor until the orbit laterally.

3. A standard coronal incision at the vertex of the scalp is made to start harvesting the pericranial flap. It would be advisable to be careful with the superficial temporal artery. This artery runs 16.68 mm in front of the tragus and divides into frontal and temporal branches above the zygomatic arch in 74% of specimens.[23]
4. It is important to make the incision from one ear to the other to improve the mobility of the superficial layers of the scalp and facilitate the harvest of the pericranial flap and help its introduction into the nasal cavity. At the level of the temporal line, the incision has to continue down until the superficial layer of the deep temporal fascia, which is continuous with the periosteal layer of the cranium.[15,21]
5. If additional length of the pericranial flap posterior to the coronal incision is needed, care must be taken in making the coronal incision to ensure that the pericranium is not divided. Extend the incision down between galeal layer and loose areolar tissue, and identify this plane of dissection.
6. Scalp incisions can be made using electrocautery, which is associated with decreased operative times and reduced blood loss, and without increased complications such as alopecia, infection, and dehiscence of the incisions.[24]
7. Dissect down along the skull and elevate the galeal fascia and the subcutaneous tissue anteriorly. This dissection is superficial to the loose areolar tissue that is a component of the pericranial flap.[15]
8. As it is explained in the section of anatomy, one must be careful at the level of the orbital rim because the deep branches of the SO and the ST arteries could arise from these main trunks 1 cm above the orbital rim. To prevent injury of these neurovascular pedicles, it is highly recommended that dissecting the first centimeter above the orbital rim is avoided.[17]
9. Posteriorly the periosteum is incised according to the tissue required for a complete closure of septal perforation. Laterally it is incised along the temporal lines. Later on, the pericranial flap is elevated to approximately 1 cm above the SO rims. Care must be taken not to damage the deep branches of the SO and ST arteries, as previously explained.[15,21]
10. The flap is folded back on itself, in its most distal area, for greater thickness of new nasal septum, suturing with dissolvable stitches (▶ Fig. 21.2).
11. The upper margin of the frontal sinus was localized through sinus transillumination; then the anterior plate of the upper portion of the frontal sinus was drilled to ensure a 30-mm width and 10-mm height frontal osteotomy. We recommend not making a

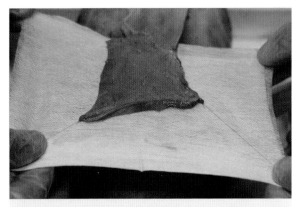

Fig. 21.2 This picture shows how to fold back the flap on itself to maximize the thickness of new nasal septum and how to mark the extremes of the flap with stitches to facilitate insertion into the nasal cavity.

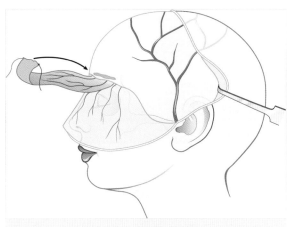

Fig. 21.4 Schematic demonstration of how to introduce pericranial flap into frontal osteotomy and how to mark the different extremes of the flap with stitches of different colors to avoid rotating the flap once inserted into the frontal sinus.

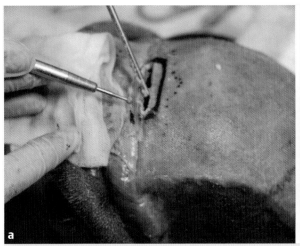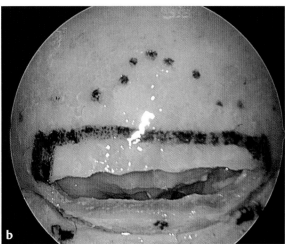

Fig. 21.3 (a) The picture shows how we drill the osteotomy of the frontal sinus. (b) The picture shows a frontal view of this osteotomy. The points mark the outline of the frontal sinus.

small osteotomy to avoid causing vascularity problems in the flap in its introduction (▶ Fig. 21.3).

12. With an endoscopic view, the pericranial flap would be introduced into the nasal cavity through the osteotomy of the frontal sinus and rotated laterally 90 degrees to be in a sagittal plane like the nasal septum. Before that, it would be advisable to mark the extremes of the flap with stitches to facilitate insertion into the nasal (▶ Fig. 21.2, ▶ Fig. 21.4).

13. The flap is sutured anteriorly to the edge of the perforation and inferiorly to the mucosa of the floor of the nasal cavity with absorbable stitches. In its most posterior portion, a suture passing through the soft palate is performed. It is anchored to the sphenoid rostrum with two stitches that pass through two holes made in the sphenoid rostrum, above the choana, thus creating a new septum made of two

layers of pericranial flap (▶ Fig. 21.5, ▶ Fig. 21.6, ▶ Fig. 21.7, ▶ Fig. 21.8).

It would be advisable to place nasal packing during 48 to 72 hours, as well as silicone nasal splints anchored in the most anterior region of the remains of the nasal septum.

21.5 Complications and Technical Solutions

As there is a lack of details about this novel pericranium flap, there is no complication described in the literature on the use of pericranial for closing a septal perforation flap.[13] However, there are some complications described in the use of pericranial flap for skull-base reconstruction,

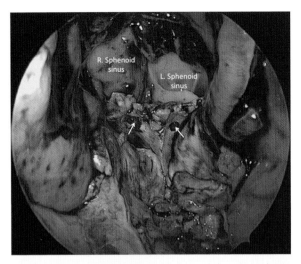

Fig. 21.5 View of total septal perforation and the sphenoid rostrum with the holes needed to anchor the pericranial flap in its posterior portion. Real case.

and most of these complications can be applied to our purpose.

- *Flap necrosis*: It is one of the most serious complications. The dissection near the orbital rim should be handled with extreme care to avoid injury to the deep branches of the SO and the ST arteries.[17] Also, the introduction into the nasal cavity and the posterior manipulation to close the perforation should be done carefully so as not to rotate the pedicle and disrupt the blood supply.
- *Injury to the frontal branch of the facial nerve*: The frontal branch of the facial nerve travels within or just deep to the superficial temporal fascia. To protect the motor innervation of the forehead, it would be advisable to elevate the frontal branch of the facial nerve within the galea when it is dissected laterally.[25]
- *Alopecia*: It is a common complication especially along the incision line. Although it is not a major complication in young males, it would be advisable to place the incision near the vertex to avoid future problems with hair loss.[15]

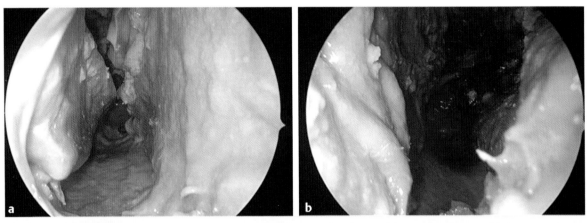

Fig. 21.6 (a) The picture shows the right side of the nasal fossa with a complete closure of the septal perforation. (b) The picture shows the same on the left side of the nasal fossa.

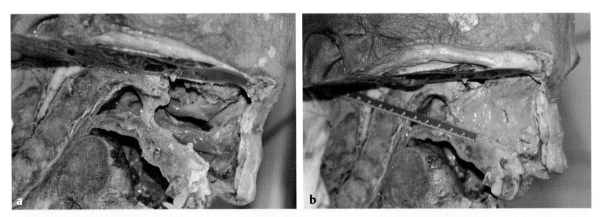

Fig. 21.7 (a) The picture shows the total septal perforation in a cadaveric specimen. (b) The picture shows the closure of this perforation with the pericranial flap.

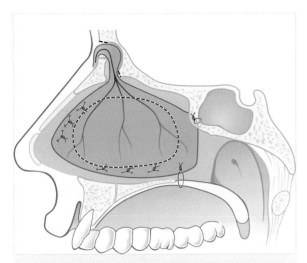

Fig. 21.8 Schematic demonstration of how to close the nasal septal perforation, by introducing the pericranial flap into the frontal sinus osteotomy. The edges of the perforation were anchored to the flap with stitches in its anterior portion and to the sphenoid rostrum with two stitches in two holes just above the choana.

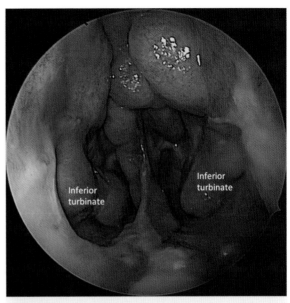

Fig. 21.9 View of a total septal perforation before the reconstruction. Real case.

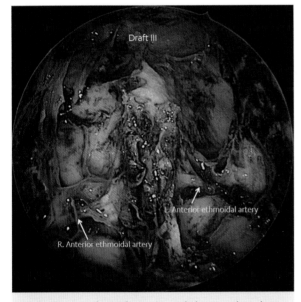

Fig. 21.10 View of a Draf type III, needed to introduce the pericranial flap. Real case.

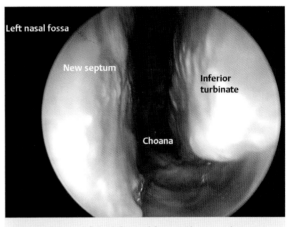

Fig. 21.11 View of the left nasal fossa with a complete reconstruction with a pericranial flap. The new septum has healed. Real case.

21.6 Case Example

We report the case of a 43-year-old man, with crusting and nasal blockage. At the physical examination we saw a near-total septal perforation (> 4 cm) (▶ Fig. 21.9). The cause of the perforation was cocaine abuse; however, at the time of exploration, the patient had spent more than

5 years without consuming cocaine. Draf type III (▶ Fig. 21.10), holes in the rostrum sphenoidale (▶ Fig. 21.11), and complete reconstruction of the nasal septum with a pericranial flap was performed, with the technique described previously (see ▶ Fig. 21.5, ▶ Fig. 21.6, ▶ Fig. 21.7, ▶ Fig. 21.8). We observed no complications 6 months after the surgery. The nasal cavity was completely healed without crusting. The new septum had enough thickness, stability, and does not vibrate with breathing (see ▶ Fig. 21.11). The previous symptoms were resolved completely with the surgery.

21.7 Tips and Tricks

Most of the tricks and recommendations have been described previously; however, it would be advisable to emphasize:

- Dissect the first centimeter above the orbits may increase the risk of flap necrosis.
- Dissect until the level of the superficial layer of the deep temporal fascia in the temporal area, to avoid the injury to the superficial temporal artery.
- Fold the pericranial flap on itself to improve its thickness.
- Suture the extremes of the flap with stitches of different colors to facilitate its introduction.
- No make a small osteotomy, it could injury the vascularity of the flap.

References

[1] Wolfe SA. The utility of pericranial flaps. Ann Plast Surg. 1978; 1(2): 147–153

[2] Tolhurst DE, Carstens MH, Greco RJ, Hurwitz DJ. The surgical anatomy of the scalp. Plast Reconstr Surg. 1991; 87(4):603–612, discussion 613–614

[3] Argenta LC, Friedman RJ, Dingman RO, Duus EC. The versatility of pericranial flaps. Plast Reconstr Surg. 1985; 76(5):695–702

[4] McCutcheon IE, Blacklock JB, Weber RS, et al. Anterior transcranial (craniofacial) resection of tumors of the paranasal sinuses: surgical technique and results. Neurosurgery. 1996; 38(3):471–479, discussion 479–480

[5] Smith JE, Ducic Y. The versatile extended pericranial flap for closure of skull base defects. Otolaryngol Head Neck Surg. 2004; 130(6):704–711

[6] Parhiscar A, Har-El G. Frontal sinus obliteration with the pericranial flap. Otolaryngol Head Neck Surg. 2001; 124(3):304–307

[7] Newman J, Costantino P, Moche J. The use of unilateral pericranial flaps for the closure of difficult medial orbital and upper lateral nasal defects. Skull Base. 2003; 13(4):205–209

[8] Moshaver A, Harris JR, Seikaly H. Use of anteriorly based pericranial flap in frontal sinus obliteration. Otolaryngol Head Neck Surg. 2006; 135(3):413–416

[9] Al-Qattan MM. The use of multifolded pericranial flaps as "plugs" and "pads.". Plast Reconstr Surg. 2001; 108(2):336–342

[10] Leatherbarrow B, Watson A, Wilcsek G. Use of the pericranial flap in medial canthal reconstruction: another application for this versatile flap. Ophthal Plast Reconstr Surg. 2006; 22(6):414–419

[11] Yoon SH, Burm JS, Yang WY, Kang SY. Vascularized bipedicled pericranial flaps for reconstruction of chronic scalp ulcer occurring after cranioplasty. Arch Plast Surg. 2013; 40(4):341–347

[12] Patel V, Osborne S, Morley AM, Malhotra R. The use of pericranial flaps for reconstruction and elevation of the lower eyelid. Orbit. 2010; 29(1):1–6

[13] Paloma V, Samper A, Cervera-Paz FJ. Surgical technique for reconstruction of the nasal septum: the pericranial flap. Head Neck. 2000; 22(1):90–94

[14] Keleş B, Oztürk K, Ciçekçibaşı AE, Büyükmumcu M. Reconstruction of large nasal septal perforations with a three layer galeal pericranial flap: an anatomical and technical study. Kulak Burun Bogaz Ihtis Derg. 2010; 20(6):293–298

[15] Carrau RL. Pericranial flap. Anatomical landmarks for endoscopic approaches to the paranasal sinuses and the skull base: Instructional Step-by-Step Dissection Guide. Alobid I, Bernal-Sprekelsen M. Ed. Thieme. 2016; In press

[16] McMinn RMH, ed. Last's Anatomy: Regional and Applied. 9th ed. London, UK: Churchill Livingstone; 1994

[17] Yoshioka N, Rhoton AL, Jr. Vascular anatomy of the anteriorly based pericranial flap. Neurosurgery. 2005; 57(1) Suppl:11–16, discussion 11–16

[18] Erdogmus S, Govsa F. Anatomy of the supraorbital region and the evaluation of it for the reconstruction of facial defects. J Craniofac Surg. 2007; 18(1):104–112

[19] Saran S, Mohandas Rao KG, Saran S, Somayaji S, N, Ashwini LS.. Morphological and morphometric analysis of supraorbital foramen and supraorbital notch: a study on dry human skulls. Oman Med J. 2012; 27(2):129–133

[20] Christensen KN, Lachman N, Pawlina W, Baum CL. Cutaneous depth of the supraorbital nerve: a cadaveric anatomic study with clinical applications to dermatology. Dermatol Surg. 2014; 40(12):1342–1348

[21] Patel MR, Shah RN, Snyderman CH, et al. Pericranial flap for endoscopic anterior skull-base reconstruction: clinical outcomes and radioanatomic analysis of preoperative planning. Neurosurgery. 2010; 66(3):506–512, discussion 512

[22] Draf W. Endonasal micro-endoscopic frontal sinus surgery: the fulda concept. Oper Tech Otolaryngol-Head Neck Surg. 1991; 2:234–240

[23] Pinar YA, Govsa F. Anatomy of the superficial temporal artery and its branches: its importance for surgery. Surg Radiol Anat. 2006; 28(3):248–253

[24] Nitta N, Fukami T, Nozaki K. Electrocautery skin incision for neurosurgery procedures—technical note. Neurol Med Chir (Tokyo). 2011; 51(1):88–91

[25] Palmer JN, Chiu AG. Atlas of endoscopic sinus and skull base surgery. In: Adelson RT, Wei C, Palmer JN, eds. Frontal Sinus Fractures. Philadelphia, PA: Elsevier; 2013:337–356

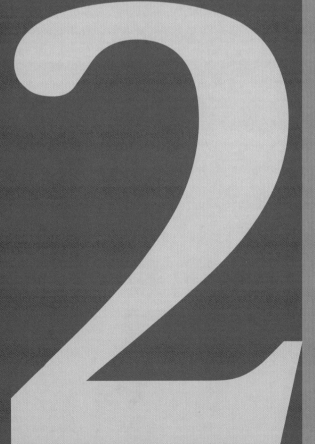
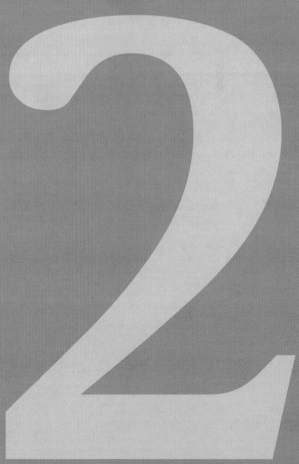

Chapter 22

Quality of Life

22 Quality of Life

Fabio Ferreli, Paolo Castelnuovo

Summary

The three-layer nasoseptal defect is a relatively rare condition, with a prevalence rate of 0.9%.[1,2] Nasal septal perforations (NSPs) give rise to not only disintegration of the septum anatomy but also impairment in normal nasal physiology.[3] Anatomical and physiologic changes following perforation lead to many different symptoms, such as sensation of nasal obstruction, crusting, epistaxis, dryness, rhinorrhea, snoring and whistling sounds, cacosmia, and headaches.[4] If these symptoms persist despite specific medical nasal care, a surgical NSP closure, if technically possible, is desirable.

For the success of a standard surgical procedure but not only technical, positive changes in quality of life should be taken into consideration. Often, the success of these surgical techniques is usually equated to anatomical closure of the perforation, while aspects related to the quality of life are not always investigated. Surgical approaches should aim to solve both the anatomical and physiologic problems of NSP. It is important to quantify surgical outcomes with objective and subjective tests and compare them with preoperative findings. Especially after rhinologic surgeries (septoplasty, rhinoplasty, conchal surgery, etc.), there can be a divergence between the objective and subjective findings.[5]

22.1 Objective Assessment

Even though relief in subjective symptoms of patients is important, an objective measurement of nasal physiology should be performed. Applying an objective assessment of pre- and postoperative nasal septal and nasal cavity physiology provides an opportunity to compare the physiologic results of various surgical procedures and can lead to the identification of the ideal method. Rhinomanometry (RMM) tests nasal airway resistance by measuring nasal airflow and the pressure produced by nasal airflow.[6] RMM has been used for the evaluation of various nasal surgical techniques.[7] Studies based on computational fluid dynamic simulations were able to show airflow patterns, temperature, and humidity distribution in nose models of healthy noses. In nose models with septal perforation, several pathological conditions could be shown. Disturbed airflow patterns mainly in the area of the posterior margin of the septal perforation are responsible for the crusting in this region. Huge vortices cause subjective nasal obstruction in patients with septal perforation. NSPs are frequently located in the anterior caudal cartilaginous part of the septum after previous surgery and cause more

symptoms than the NSPs, which are located more in the cranial or more in the posterior portion.[8]

In fact, most of the symptomatic NSPs are in the anterior portion of the septum, whereas posterior septal defects can be asymptomatic. Knowledge regarding the temperature and humidity profile within septal perforation is scarce. Lindemann et al performed two in vivo studies to investigate these parameters comparing healthy volunteers and patients with NSP as well as before and after surgical closure of NSP. They observed a significantly reduced increase in humidity in patients with NSP compared to the healthy volunteers. The patients with NSP suffered significantly more from nasal dryness. Postoperatively, the increase in temperature and humidity was significantly higher than preoperatively.[9]

Olfaction has an important role in the human interaction with the environment, and changes in olfaction abilities due to NSP can lead to a significant decrease in quality of life. The surgical repair of nasal septal perforation is known to improve nasal respiratory airflow, which seems to be beneficial to the patient's olfactory abilities. However, there are only limited data on the effect of nasal septal perforation closure on olfaction, and most studies reported contradictory results.[10,11,12] In a recent study, Altun and Hanci reported a statistically significant improvement in olfactory function determined by using the Sniffin' Sticks on the short- and long-term olfactory abilities of 42 patients with NSP after surgical repair.[13]

22.2 Subjective Assessment

There are a limited number of studies referring to symptom control in patients with NSP who receive surgical treatments.[4]

Subjective clinical evaluations following nasal surgery can be assessed with different scoring charts. Currently, there are several validated assessments for general quality of life as well as for sinonasal conditions.[14,15,16,17] The Nasal Obstruction Symptom Evaluation (NOSE) is one of the most highly used scoring systems.[14]

Ozturk et al showed a correlation between the symptom control, evaluated by NOSE, and improvements in nasal physiology, confirmed by rhinomanometric measurements.[18] There are also special assessments for sinonasal complaints; among them are the "Nasal Symptom Questionnaire', 'Rhino-Sinusitis Disability Index', "General Nasal Patient Inventory," 'Rhinosinusitis Quality of Life Survey," and "Sino-Nasal Outcome Test 20."[15,16,17,19,20,21]

The Glasgow Benefit Inventory (GBI) is especially designed for ENT (ear-nose-throat) health problems and procedures. Introduced in 1996, this survey is composed of 18 questions and reflects changes in health conditions after surgical or conservative treatments. Health status is defined as the general perception of one's own health, including all psychosocial, social, and physical aspects. The SNOT-20 is a shortened form of the Rhinosinusitis Outcome Measure (RSOM-31) introduced by Piccirillo et al,[21] containing general and rhinosinusitis-related questions. The SNOT-20 queries 20 symptoms of rhinosinusitis that are divided into five subgroups: nasal, paranasal, sleeping, social, and emotional. In 2008, Baumann introduced a slightly altered German version of the SNOT-20: The Sino-Nasal Outcome Test 20 German Adapted Version (SNOT-20 GAV). To the SNOT-20 GAV, the subscores primary nasal symptoms, secondary rhinogenic symptoms, and general quality of life were added to facilitate a more specific evaluation. To evaluate quality of life in patients following closure of a nasoseptal defect via obturator, the 20 questions on the SNOT-20 GAV were expanded to include five nasoseptal defect-specific questions introduced by Neumann in 2010 regarding bleeding, whistling noise, pain, temperature perception, and foreign-body sensation (SNOT-20 GAV SDT).[22] These two questionnaires (GBI and SNOT-20 GAV) were combined to cover all four dimensions of patients' health-related quality of life (psychosomatic, functional, social, and psychological-emotional). The *psychosomatic dimension* (pain, nasal breathing impairment, nosebleeds) is well represented by Neumann's expanded version of the SNOT 20 GAV SDT. The *functional dimension* (daily life activities) and *social dimension* (family relationships and friendships) are included in the 18 questions in the GBI. The *psychological-emotional dimension* (regarding fear, depression, and sadness) is reflected both in the GBI and SNOT 20 GAV SDT. Thus both the GBI and SNOT 20 GAV SDT fulfill the assessment requirement of reflecting at least three of the four dimensions. In the study of Bast et al, the GBI and SNOT-20GAV SDT, with septal defect-specific items, were used to evaluate the quality of life following surgical septal perforation closure.[23] The evaluation of the GBI yielded a significant improvement for the total score and subscore "general health," showing a positive change in the quality of life of patients following a surgical septum closure. To investigate specific changes in symptoms through surgical interventions on the nasal septum or nasal cavities, the SNOT 20 GAV SDT was evaluated. The significant reduction in the total score, the subscore "primary nasal symptoms," and "septum-specific symptoms" not only shows that the rhinogenic condition generally improved, but also that defect-specific symptoms were significantly reduced.[23] Finally, NSP results in a double-sided problem: anatomical and physiologic. Surgical approaches should address both of these issues. The application of subjective and objective tests during the pre- and postoperative period will help surgeons assess the applied techniques. In past studies, the success of a surgical approach has been represented only by the closure rate. The closing of the NSP only deals with anatomical aspects of the problem. Besides the anatomical defect, NSP results in impairments of nasal physiology. The success of a medical or surgical intervention is determined by not only the technical success of the procedure but also positive changes in patients' quality of life. More recent studies show as a successful NSP surgical closure leads not only to a significant improvement in perforation-specific and primary nasal symptoms but also to an improvement in general health and therefore to a subjectively improved quality of life.

References

[1] Watson D, Barkdull G. Surgical management of the septal perforation. Otolaryngol Clin North Am. 2009; 42(3):483–493

[2] Stange T, Schultz-Coulon HJ. [Closure of nasoseptal defects in Germany: the current state of the art][in German]. Laryngorhinootologie. 2010; 89(3):157–161

[3] Leong SC, Chen XB, Lee HP, Wang DY. A review of the implications of computational fluid dynamic studies on nasal airflow and physiology. Rhinology. 2010; 48(2):139–145

[4] Cogswell LK, Goodacre TE. The management of nasoseptal perforation. Br J Plast Surg. 2000; 53(2):117–120

[5] Sipilä J, Suonpää J. A prospective study using rhinomanometry and patient clinical satisfaction to determine if objective measurements of nasal airway resistance can improve the quality of septoplasty. Eur Arch Otorhinolaryngol. 1997; 254(8):387–390

[6] Clement PA. Committee report on standardization of rhinomanometry. Rhinology. 1984; 22(3):151–155

[7] Broms P, Jonson B, Malm L. Rhinomanometry. IV. A pre- and postoperative evaluation in functional septoplasty. Acta Otolaryngol. 1982; 94(5–6):523–529

[8] Lindemann J, Reichert M, Kroger R, Schulder P, Hoffman T, Sommer F. Numerical simulation of humidification and heating during inspiration in nose models with three different located septal perforations. Eur Arch Otorhinolaryngol. 2015

[9] Lindemann J, Leiacker R, Stehmer V, Rettinger G, Keck T. Intranasal temperature and humidity profile in patients with nasal septal perforation before and after surgical closure. Clin Otolaryngol Allied Sci. 2001; 26(5):433–437

[10] Fyrmpas G, Tsalighopoulos M, Constantinidis J. Lateralized olfactory difference in patients with a nasal septal deviation before and after septoplasty. Hippokratia. 2012; 16(2):166–169

[11] Pfaar O, Hüttenbrink KB, Hummel T. Assessment of olfactory function after septoplasty: a longitudinal study. Rhinology. 2004; 42(4):195–199

[12] Faramarzi M, Baradaranfar MH, Abouali O, et al. Numerical investigation of the flow field in realistic nasal septal perforation geometry. Allergy Rhinol (Providence). 2014; 5(2):70–77

[13] Altun H, Hanci D. Olfaction improvement after nasal septal perforation repair with the "cross-stealing" technique. Am J Rhinol Allergy. 2015; 29(5):e142–e145

[14] Stewart MG, Witsell DL, Smith TL, Weaver EM, Yueh B, Hannley MT. Development and validation of the Nasal Obstruction Symptom Evaluation (NOSE) scale. Otolaryngol Head Neck Surg. 2004; 130(2):157–163

[15] Baumann I. [Validated instruments to measure quality of life in patients with chronic rhinosinusitis]. HNO. 2009; 57(9):873–881

[16] Fahmy FF, McCombe A, Mckiernan DC. Sino nasal assessment questionnaire, a patient focused, rhinosinusitis specific outcome measure. Rhinology. 2002; 40(4):195–197

[17] Baumann I, Plinkert PK, De Maddelena H. [Development of a grading scale for the Sino-Nasal Outcome Test-20 German Adapted Version (SNOT-20 GAV)][in German]. HNO. 2008; 56(8):784–788

[18] Ozturk S, Zor F, Ozturk S, Kartal O, Alhan D, Isik S. A new approach to objective evaluation of the success of nasal septum perforation. Arch Plast Surg. 2014; 41(4):403–406

[19] Robinson K, Gatehouse S, Browning GG. Measuring patient benefit from otorhinolaryngological surgery and therapy. Ann Otol Rhinol Laryngol. 1996; 105(6):415–422

[20] Neumann A, Lehmann N, Stange T, et al. [Patients' satisfaction after nasal septal and turbinate surgery. Results of a questionnaire][in German]. Laryngorhinootologie. 2007; 86(10):706–713

[21] Piccirillo JF, Merritt MG, Jr, Richards ML. Psychometric and clinimetric validity of the 20-Item Sino-Nasal Outcome Test (SNOT-20). Otolaryngol Head Neck Surg. 2002; 126(1):41–47

[22] Neumann A, Schneider M, Tholen C, Minovi A. [Inoperable nasoseptal defects: closure with custom-made Silastic prostheses][in German]. HNO. 2010; 58(4):364–370

[23] Bast F, Heimer A, Schrom T. Surgical closure of nasoseptal defects: postoperative patient satisfaction. ORL J Otorhinolaryngol Relat Spec. 2012; 74(6):299–303

Chapter 23

Endoscopic Repair for Septal Perforation: Algorithm

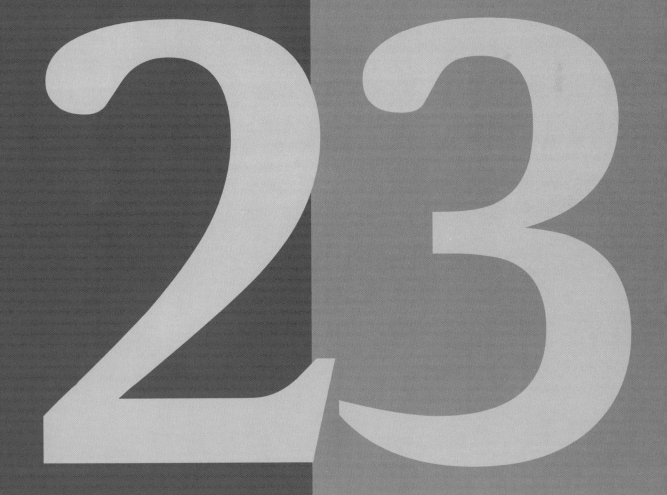

23 Endoscopic Repair for Septal Perforation: Algorithm

Fabio Ferreli, Paolo Castelnuovo

23.1 Introduction

Nasal septal perforation (NSP) repair remains a challenging issue for rhinologists—not only due to its technical aspects but also in choosing the most suitable approach concerning the specific nasal anatomic situation in addition to the surgeon's experience.

The goal should be to provide a closure for the NSP without tension, restore the normal intranasal function, and, in some cases, to reconstruct the nasal support.

NSPs are usually an incidental finding in asymptomatic patients during physical examination. If there are no complaints, no treatment is necessary, and when the perforation causes only mild symptoms, conservative management can be attempted at first, such as nasal irrigation with isotonic saline and/or antibiotic ointment.

If complaints persist despite nonsurgical therapy, surgery should then be considered. Although many surgical techniques for the repair of NSP have been attempted for many decades, no agreement has yet been reached on the most suitable method for the best outcome.

NSP can be repaired with different approaches, such as external rhinoplasty, intranasal (endoscopic or microscopic), sublabial, and midfacial degloving.[1]

A literature review published in 2007 did not make any significant conclusion regarding the relative rate of success for the various techniques used to close NSP.[1]

Over the last decade, a wide variety of endoscopic endonasal approaches (EEAs) have been described for the treatment of NSP. Case series and case reports showing favorable outcomes via an EEA have recently increased despite its technical difficulties, particularly in cases of small to moderate perforations by the benefit of the endoscopic technique.[2,3,4,5,6,7,8,9,10,11,12,13,14,15]

Depending on the size of the perforation and nasal anatomic condition, treatment method and flap choice may differ. This chapter provides a decisional algorithm on different endoscopic techniques regarding several local aspects (e.g., size and location of the defect, previous septal surgery).

23.2 Relevant Analytical Factors

NSPs located in the posterior part of the septum tend to be asymptomatic, whereas anterior perforations often present symptoms (e.g., crusting, a sensation of nasal obstruction, bleeding, headache, dryness, and whistling); thus we considered only the latter as candidates for surgery.

Measuring the size of the perforation preoperatively is an important factor for planning the operation; however, the size usually increases with elevation of mucoperichondrial flap and trimming margins.

According to current literature, NSP may be stratified based on size as follows: small perforations 0.5 cm or less, medium perforations between 0.5 and 2 cm, large perforations greater than 2 cm.

Although defects larger than 2 cm in length are generally accepted as a large size, the upper limit of small size differs between authors, up to 0.5 or 1 cm.[16,17]

Computed tomographic (CT) scan of the paranasal sinus is an evaluation tool used not only to measure the septum defect but also to evaluate the amount of residual bone/cartilage.

In NSPs that have occurred after septoplasty, there is usually very little cartilage left, and this makes dissection of the flaps more difficult.

For small- to middle-sized NSP, different techniques require a nasal septum with a residual underlying cartilage or bone, which help perform a meticulous dissection to elevate the mucoperichondrium-mucoperiostium.[2,3,4,5,13,14]

For these types of techniques, which use mucoperichondrial and mucoperiosteal septal tissue to close the perforation, the amount of septal structures remains as fundamental prognostic indicator of successful surgery.

Therefore, when it is not possible to perform an easy dissection of the septal mucosa, it is preferable to choose alternative techniques that use mucosal flaps harvested in other anatomical areas.[6,7,8,9]

It is also important to check the quality of the intranasal anatomical structures preoperatively, which represented potential donor sites of grafts or flaps (inferior turbinate, middle turbinate, floor of the nasal fossa). Several local or regional flaps have been described for closure of septal perforations, but in our opinion, only the techniques adopting nasal mucosal flaps achieve normal nasal physiology because they use the normal respiratory epithelium for closure.

Small to moderate perforations can be repaired with local advancement flaps alone or combined with interposition grafts. Some centers have reported good outcome without interposition grafts, and the promising results show that the need for an interposition graft has not been established yet.[13,14,15,18]

Nevertheless, according to different case series outcomes, in small and medium perforations (<2 cm), the interposition of a graft between the two mucosal layers is, in our opinion, useless.

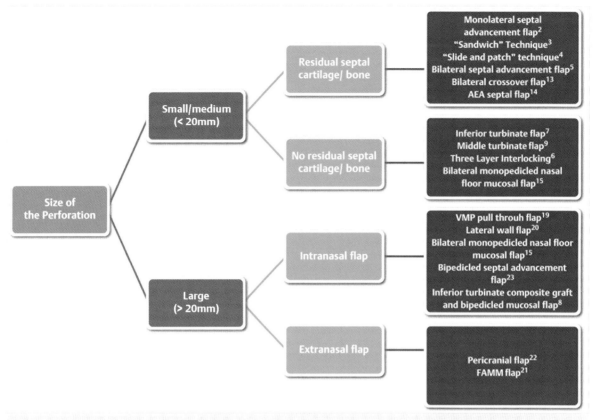

Fig. 23.1 Proposed algorithm for surgical endoscopic or endoscopic-assisted repair of nasal septal perforations. AEA, anterior ethmoidal artery; FAMM, facial artery musculomucosal; VMP, vascularized mucoperiosteal

A recent systematic review found that interposition grafts appeared to help closure, as a template for mucosal migration during the healing process, but this factor was not considered statistically significant.[16] About the necessity for bilateral flap provision, unilateral flap coverage was advocated by some authors, as it limits the donor area to one side of the nose, and thus preserves more nasal respiratory mucosa while achieving favorable closure rates.[2,3,4,5,6,7,8,9,10,11,12,13,14] Even in patients with moderate to large perforation, complete closure can be obtained by applying a unilateral well-vascularized mucoperiosteal flap.[19]

Large perforations with previous history of extensive septal trauma or surgery, however, cartilaginous remnants are usually insufficient and their quality can be quite low. In this situation, it is better to use mucosal flaps harvested in other anatomic sites (lateral nasal wall flap, facial artery musculomucosal flap, pericranial flap)[20,21,22] and adopt autologous graft materials to reconstruct the nasal support; for example, conchal cartilage is a good option if septal cartilage is not available.[6,23]

We propose this algorithm for the endoscopic endonasal techniques for NSP repair (► Fig. 23.1).

References

[1] Goh AY, Hussain SS. Different surgical treatments for nasal septal perforation and their outcomes. J Laryngol Otol. 2007; 121(5):419–426

[2] Lee HR, Ahn DB, Park JH, et al. Endoscopic repairment of septal perforation with using a unilateral nasal mucosal flap. Clin Exp Otorhinolaryngol. 2008; 1(3):154–157

[3] Chen FH, Rui X, Deng J, Wen YH, Xu G, Shi JB. Endoscopic sandwich technique for moderate nasal septal perforations. Laryngoscope. 2012; 122(11):2367–2372

[4] Cassano M. Endoscopic repair of nasal septal perforation with "slide and patch" technique. Otolaryngol Head Neck Surg. 2014; 151(1):176–178

[5] Tasca I, Compadretti GC. Closure of nasal septal perforation via endonasal approach. Otolaryngol Head Neck Surg. 2006; 135(6):922–927

[6] Kaya E, Cingi C, Olgun Y, Soken H, Pinarbasli Ö. Three layer interlocking: a novel technique for repairing a nasal septum perforation. Ann Otol Rhinol Laryngol. 2015; 124(3):212–215

[7] Friedman M, Ibrahim H, Ramakrishnan V. Inferior turbinate flap for repair of nasal septal perforation. Laryngoscope. 2003; 113(8):1425–1428

[8] Tastan E, Aydogan F, Aydin E, et al. Inferior turbinate composite graft for repair of nasal septal perforation. Am J Rhinol Allergy. 2012; 26 (3):237–242

[9] Hanci D, Altun H. Repair of nasal septal perforation using middle turbinate flap (monopedicled superiorly based bone included conchal flap): a new unilateral middle turbinate mucosal flap technique. Eur Arch Otorhinolaryngol. 2015; 272(7):1707–1712

[10] Kazkayasi M, Tuna E, Kilic C. Bullous middle turbinate flap for the repair of nasal septal perforation. J Otolaryngol Head Neck Surg. 2010; 39(2):203–206

[11] Hier MP, Yoskovitch A, Panje WR. Endoscopic repair of a nasal septal perforation. J Otolaryngol. 2002; 31(5):323–326

[12] Kazkayasi M, Yalcinozan ET. Uncinate process in the repair of naso-septal perforation. Aesthetic Plast Surg. 2011; 35(5):878–881

[13] Pignatari S, Nogueira JF, Stamm AC. Endoscopic "crossover flap" technique for nasal septal perforations. Otolaryngol Head Neck Surg. 2010; 142(1):132–134.e1

[14] Castelnuovo P, Ferreli F, Khodaei I, Palma P. Anterior ethmoidal artery septal flap for the management of septal perforation. Arch Facial Plast Surg. 2011; 13(6):411–414

[15] Presutti L, Alicandri Ciufelli M, Marchioni D, Villari D, Marchetti A, Mattioli F. Nasal septal perforations: our surgical technique. Otolaryngol Head Neck Surg. 2007; 136(3):369–372

[16] Kim SW, Rhee CS. Nasal septal perforation repair: predictive factors and systematic review of the literature. Curr Opin Otolaryngol Head Neck Surg. 2012; 20(1):58–65

[17] Watson D, Barkdull G. Surgical management of the septal perforation. Otolaryngol Clin North Am. 2009; 42(3):483–493

[18] Teymoortash A, Werner JA. Repair of nasal septal perforation using a simple unilateral inferior meatal mucosal flap. J Plast Reconstr Aesthet Surg. 2009; 62(10):1261–1264

[19] Shikowitz MJ. Vascularized mucoperiosteal pull through flap for closure of large septal perforation: a new technique. Laryngoscope. 2007; 117(4):750–755

[20] Alobid I, Mason E, Solares CA, et al. Pedicled lateral nasal wall flap for the reconstruction of the nasal septum perforation. A radio-anatomical study. Rhinology. 2015; 53(3):235–241

[21] Heller JB, Gabbay JS, Trussler A, Heller MM, Bradley JP. Repair of large nasal septal perforations using facial artery musculomucosal (FAMM) flap. Ann Plast Surg. 2005; 55(5):456–459

[22] Paloma V, Samper A, Cervera-Paz FJ. Surgical technique for reconstruction of the nasal septum: the pericranial flap. Head Neck. 2000; 22(1):90–94

[23] Giacomini PG, Ferraro S, Di Girolamo S, Ottaviani F. Large nasal septal perforation repair by closed endoscopically assisted approach. Ann Plast Surg. 2011; 66(6):633–636

Index